Diagnostic Function Tests in Chemical Pathology

Diagnostic Function Tests in Chemical Pathology

by

P. T. Lascelles MD, FRCPath

Honorary Consultant in Chemical Pathology,
The National Hospitals for Nervous Diseases,
Queen Square and Maida Vale,
London

and

D. Donaldson MB, ChB, MRCP, FRCPath

Consultant in Chemical Pathology,
East Surrey Hospital, Redhill, Surrey,
and Crawley Hospital, Crawley,
West Sussex

KLUWER ACADEMIC PUBLISHERS
DORDRECHT / BOSTON / LONDON

Distributors

for the United States and Canada: Kluwer Academic Publishers, PO Box 358, Accord Station, Hingham, MA 02018-0358, USA
for all other countries: Kluwer Academic Publishers Group, Distribution Center, PO Box 322, 3300 AH Dordrecht, The Netherlands

British Library Cataloguing in Publication Data

Lascelles, P.T
    Diagnostic funtion tests in chemical pathology.
    1. Medicine. Diagnosis. Tests
    I. Title II. Donaldson, D.
    616.07'5

    ISBN 0-7462-0108-7
    ISBN 0-7462-0107-9 pbk

Copyright

Published in the United Kingdom by Kluwer Academic Publishers, PO Box 55, Lancaster, UK.

Kluwer Academic Publishers BV incorporates the publishing programmes of D. Reidel, Martinus Nijhoff, Dr W. Junk and MTP Press.

Lasertypeset by Martin Lister Publishing Services, Carnforth, Lancashire
Printed in Great Britain by Redwood Burn Ltd, Trowbridge, Wiltshire, UK

Contents

Contents

Contents

Preface

This book is written for hospital doctors, nurses, biochemists, medical laboratory scientific officers and phlebotomists involved with the biochemical investigation of patients. It is hoped, also, that general practitioners and medical students will find it of help.

Whilst the vast majority of biochemical tests assess the level of constituents in blood and urine at a given point in time, an important additional parameter is the assessment of physiological reserve function by means of loading tests, prolonged fasting, exercise and clearance studies. The protocol and interpretation of response of each of these stress tests form the main basis of the text. An attempt has been made to be reasonably comprehensive in the range of tests described; hence, not only have some rather older ones been retained, but also some very recently introduced ones included. It is appreciated that practice varies widely from laboratory to laboratory with respect to protocol, sample collection, methodology and quotation of reference ranges, and no doubt also from clinician to clinician, particularly regarding interpretation of results. In paediatric work, micromethods will demand much smaller volumes of blood than those stated here, which relate generally to adult medicine. The account, therefore, must be seen as a guide to practice rather than as a recipe; it is in no way an attempt to standardise procedures, which depend on the local requirements.

The investigations have been listed in alphabetical order, and much care has been taken to provide a comprehensive index which includes both clinical diagnoses and technical terms.

The temptation to give detailed references has been resisted, but a few selected ones have been quoted where it is felt that further reading is necessary. However, the aim of the book remains to provide an easily accessible and fairly comprehensive source of information for performing a wide range of biochemical investigations on both in-patients and out-patients.

Although every care has been taken to ensure accuracy, inevi-

ix

tably some errors are likely to creep into a text such as this. Accordingly, we are grateful to many friends and colleagues who have pointed out mistakes and who have made helpful criticisms.

Our particular gratitude goes to Mrs Marina Shaw who has so ably prepared the manuscript. We would also like to thank our publishers for their almost unbelievable forbearance during the long period taken for completion of this work and Dr R.D. Hawkins for valuable help in proof-reading.

P.T.L.

D.D.

September 1989

L-ALANINE LOAD TEST[1]

Principle

L-Alanine is transaminated to ammonia, which enters the urea cycle, thereby stimulating production of urea. An intravenous L-alanine load, followed by measurement of end-products of the urea cycle, including urinary orotic acid excretion, and calculations of the rate of urea synthesis, time of maximal urea synthesis and the kinetics of plasma ammonia, ornithine, glutamate and glutamine, permits characterisation of a minimal or latent enzyme defect in this cycle. Gross defects of the cycle will have presented already with marked basal hyperammonaemia.

Indication

This test is indicated in the families of patients suspected clinically of having an enzyme defect in the urea cycle, and also in patients with unexplained mild hyperammonaemia at any age, and particularly in the relatives of patients who have reacted unfavourably to valproate therapy by producing hyperammonaemia. **Caution: this test is contraindicated in patients with severe hyperammonaemia from any cause.**

Patient Preparation

The patient fasts overnight and throughout the test, but is encouraged to drink water (250 ml every 40 min). Smoking is not permitted.

Protocol

L-Alanine (250 mg/kg body weight), taken from a sterile 50 ml ampoule, is infused in physiological saline as a 10% w/v solution via an intravenous catheter (i.e. a concentration of 1 g L-alanine/10 ml saline) over a period of 15 min; this is equivalent to 2.5 ml of solution/kg body weight. Venous blood (2 ml) is collected into each of 2 bottles, a polythene one for plasma ammonia estimation (special collection, see Appendix III) and a glass one for measurement of serum urea, every 20 min for 2 h prior to and at the commencement of the infusion. Further samples are taken every 10 min for 1 h following the start of the infusion, every 15 min for the next 1 h and then every 20 min for a further 2 h period. An intravenous catheter, inserted 30 min prior to collection of the first

1

blood sample, should be used. The bladder is emptied 2 h prior to commencing the infusion, the urine being discarded. All further urine samples are collected at 40 min intervals separately into plain polythene bottles over the next 6 h for urea and the organic acid, orotic acid (special collection, see Appendix III), estimation.

Sample Handling

Venous blood is processed as for estimation of serum urea and plasma ammonia, and urine as for estimation of urea and organic acids.

Normal Response

Changes in the rate of urea synthesis should be within well defined limits, without hyperammonaemia, excessive orotic acid excretion, or any delay in the time of peak urea synthesis.

Interpretation

Hyperammonaemia, changed kinetics of urea synthesis and altered urinary orotic acid excretion indicate a defect in the urea cycle. Deficiency of carbamoyl phosphate synthetase is associated with decreased orotic acid excretion, whereas deficiency of ornithine carbamoyl transferase (OCT) is associated with increased orotic acid excretion. These changes, which may be latent or manifested in a mild form in carriers, are identified by this test.

Comment

The intravenous 'L-Alanine load test' provides far more sensitive and reliable information concerning prediction of a defect in the urea cycle than does either an oral L-alanine load or exposure to high dietary protein and is essentially a research tool for use in special centres. Sodium valproate in therapeutic concentration raises plasma ammonia and decreases orotic acid excretion in normal subjects by decreasing activity of the enzyme carbamoyl phosphate synthetase. However, in female subjects with mild OCT deficiency or in carriers of the enzyme defect, the effects of valproate therapy may be predominantly on this enzyme, causing hyperammonaemia and high orotic acid excretion. In such subjects this test may prove predictive of hazards from valproate administration.

AMMONIUM CHLORIDE LOAD TEST

Principle

In the commoner and more severe form of renal tubular acidosis (distal RTA, type I), there is failure of hydrogen ion (H^+) excretion by the distal renal tubules, leading to metabolic acidosis. Following administration of ammonium chloride, which dissociates into ammonia and H^+, there is an increase in the degree of acidosis, in the presence of which, failure to produce a urine pH<5.2 confirms the diagnosis. In the rarer form of renal tubular acidosis (proximal RTA, type II), there is excessive loss of bicarbonate from the proximal renal tubules, but H^+ secretion and bicarbonate generation by the cells of the distal tubules continues. If, however, the serum bicarbonate falls to a low level, then less bicarbonate reaches the distal tubules in spite of the impaired proximal tubular reabsorption. In these circumstances the H^+ produced by the distal tubules combine with phosphate and ammonia instead of bicarbonate (which is not available). Administration of ammonium chloride in this case reveals ability to form an acid urine of pH<5.2. This test does not, however, differentiate satisfactorily between these two forms of renal tubular acidosis.

Indication

This test is used to confirm the diagnosis of distal RTA (type I). **Caution: the test is dangerous and is contraindicated in any patient with a high plasma ammonia (e.g. hepatic failure) or in the presence of a defect in the urea cycle. The test should not be carried out in patients with metabolic acidosis due to any other cause (e.g. renal failure).**

Patient Preparation

The patient should receive nil by mouth for the 8 h preceding the test.

Protocol

Ammonium chloride (100 mg/kg body weight) is given orally in water over a period of 10 min. Venous blood (5 ml) is collected into a polythene bottle containing heparin before the ammonium chloride is given and again 6 h later. All urine samples are collected

3

separately into plain polythene bottles at convenient intervals for 8 h for pH measurement (special collection, see Appendix III).

Sample Handling

Blood samples are sent to the laboratory routinely for serum bicarbonate estimation. Each specimen of urine, collected individually and without addition of preservative, is dispatched immediately for measurement of pH without delay.

Normal Response

The urine pH should fall to <5.2 in at least one specimen, and the serum bicarbonate should remain unchanged.

Interpretation

In patients with proximal RTA (type II), as also in normal subjects and those with generalised renal tubular damage, the urine pH falls to <5.2 at some point during the test. In patients with distal RTA (type I), the urine pH remains above this level, at >6.0, thus indicating inability to acidify the urine in spite of a low serum bicarbonate concentration.

Comment

This is a simple and useful test.

ANTIPYRINE CLEARANCE TEST[2]

Principle

Measurements of serial plasma levels of antipyrine, following administration of a standard dose of the compound, permit calculation of its biological half-life. The latter is dependent on the degree of hepatic cytochrome P450 microsomal hydroxylation activity, which in turn reflects the extent of enzyme induction by the patient's current or recent drug medication. The antipyrine half-life thus measures the detoxification rate of the many drugs which are eliminated by liver hydroxylation, e.g. barbiturates, other anticonvulsants and oral contraceptive preparations.

Indication

This test is a research procedure used for the assessment of hepatic microsomal P450 enzyme induction under precisely defined conditions.

Patient Preparation

The patient fasts overnight and for the first 3 h of the test and should remain at rest in bed. Smoking is not permitted. The usual morning drug medication may be continued 30 min after the dose of antipyrine has been given.

Protocol

Antipyrine (18 mg/kg body weight to the nearest 100 mg) is given orally in the morning. Venous blood (10 ml) is collected into glass bottles containing heparin at 0, 1, 4, 8, 12 and 24 h after taking the antipyrine. Exact timing of the blood samples must be observed.

Sample Handling

Plasma is stored at – 20 °C for estimation of antipyrine. The test may be repeated at (say) 3 weeks after changing the drug regimen which is suspected of influencing hepatic microsomal P450 enzyme induction.

Normal Response

The half-life of antipyrine is 11.5–13.5 h in males and 10.0–12.0 h in females; in elderly subjects it is 16.5 h, but in children it is 50% of the adult value.

Interpretation

Other factors affecting the antipyrine half-life include diet (e.g. Brassica vegetables, smoked and barbecued meats), smoking, abnormal liver function and alcohol ingestion.

Comment

This is a difficult assay which is not useful as a routine procedure. Extrapolation from a given subject to others, even under defined conditions, is often not valid, but comparison in one subject (acting as his/her own control) on repeated testing is more meaningful with reference to changes in hepatic microsomal P450 enzyme induction by different drug regimens, other factors (including diet) being kept constant.

L-ARGININE INFUSION TEST

Principle

L-Arginine stimulates growth hormone (GH) release from the anterior pituitary gland. Following administration, L-arginine causes elevation of serum GH levels, measurements of which serve as a test of anterior pituitary function.

Indication

This test is used in patients suspected of having GH deficiency, e.g. children with retarded growth or adults with suspected panhypopituitarism.

Patient Preparation

The patient should be investigated under 'basal conditions' (see Appendix I), except that there is no restriction on water intake.

Protocol

L-Arginine monochloride (500 mg/kg body weight, with maximum dose being 30 g) is infused intravenously in 100 ml of physiological saline over a period of 30 min. Venous blood (5 ml) is collected at −30, 0, 30, 60, 90 and 120 min after commencing the infusion, into plain glass bottles. An intravenous catheter, inserted 30 min prior to collection of the first blood sample, should be used.

Sample Handling

This is as for serum GH estimation.

Normal Response

The serum GH level, commencing at <10 mIU/L, rises to >20 mIU/L at 30–60 min after the start of the L-arginine infusion.

Interpretation

Inadequate responses occur in GH deficiency, in primary hypothyroidism and in 15% of normal subjects. An adequate response excludes GH deficiency.

Comment

An inadequate response must be confirmed by performing other tests of pituitary function. The side effects in this test are minimal. This is only one of several factors known to increase GH release; these include Bovril, clonidine, L-dopa, glucagon and insulin.

BILE ACID BREATH TEST[3]

Principle

Glycocholic acid, like other bile acids, is normally wholly absorbed by the small intestine, the glycine portion of the molecule being metabolised to carbon dioxide (CO_2), which appears in the expired breath. If ^{14}C-glycocholic acid is administered orally, [14]CO_2 appears in the breath soon after the dose if there is excessive bacterial activity in the small intestine; however, failure of absorption of bile acids in malabsorption syndromes or after small intestinal resection results in [14]CO_2 appearing in the breath later, due to the action of normal bacteria lower down in the colon. In the latter case, significant radioactivity is also found in the faeces.

Indication

This test is of value in differentiating small bowel stasis with bacterial overgrowth from malabsorption.

Patient Preparation

The patient fasts overnight. Smoking is not permitted. The test may be performed on in-patients or out-patients.

Protocol

[14]C-Glycocholic acid (185 kBq, 5 μCi) is administered orally with a Lundh test meal (see page 105). Expired air is collected hourly for 6 h in bottles containing a trapping agent (e.g. hyamine hydroxide) and an indicator (e.g. thymolphthalein); this indicator will change from blue to colourless when sufficient CO_2 has been collected. However, it would not matter if breath collection continued beyond that point, because excess CO_2 could not be retained in solution, and would not seriously interfere with the test. Faeces are collected for 24 h.

Sample Handling

The presence of [14]CO_2 in the expired breath at 2, 4 and 6 h is expressed as a percentage of the dose of radioactivity administered; ^{14}C is measured in the faeces.

9

Normal Response

Only trace amounts of radioactivity are present in the breath at any time, or in the faeces.

Interpretation

Radioactivity in the first 3 breath samples indicates bacterial over-growth in the small intestine. Radioactivity, especially in the last 3 samples, but possibly also earlier, indicates impaired absorption of bile acids as a result of malabsorption or ileal resection/by-pass. Malabsorption is confirmed by the detection of significant radioactivity in the faeces.

Comment

This is a simple and reliable test, involving only trace amounts of radioactivity.

BOVRIL STIMULATION TEST

Principle

The high, but imprecisely known, amino acid (particularly L-arginine) content of Bovril is responsible, in children, for the release of growth hormone (GH) from the anterior pituitary gland. Following administration, Bovril causes elevation of serum GH levels, measurements of which serve as a test of anterior pituitary function.

Indication

This test is used mainly to assess GH response in children. It is sometimes used as a preliminary screening test in the assessment of adult patients suspected of having hypopituitarism.

Patient Preparation

The patient should be investigated under 'basal conditions' (see Appendix I), except that there is no restriction on water intake.

Protocol

Bovril (330 mg/kg body weight, or 14 g/m^2 body surface area) is administered orally in 10 times its volume of hot water (i.e. an approximately 10% solution w/v). Venous blood (5 ml) is collected at – 30, 0, 30, 60, 90 and 120 min after administration of Bovril, into plain glass bottles. An intravenous catheter, inserted 30 min prior to collection of the first blood sample, should be used.

Sample Handling

This is as for serum GH estimation.

Normal Response

In children with base-line serum GH levels of <10 mIU/L, there should be a rise to >20 mIU/L.

Interpretation

A normal response negates GH deficiency. Failure to demonstrate a normal GH response is suggestive of, but does not necessarily confirm, hypopituitarism; an impaired response is also seen in primary hypothyroidism, socially deprived children, and 20% of

11

normal children.

Comment

This test has latterly lost favour as a screening test. As an alternative to Bovril, exercise also provokes GH release. The 'Bovril stimulation test' is a useful and safe test in children, especially those under 10 years of age. A serum GH of >20 mIU/L 15 min after completing 15 min of vigorous exercise indicates a good response to exercise alone, and may render this test unnecessary. This is only one of several factors known to increase GH release; these include L-arginine, clonidine, L-dopa, glucagon and insulin.

BROMSULPHTHALEIN (BSP) EXCRETION TEST

Principle

Bromsulphthalein (BSP), following intravenous administration, is removed from the circulation (where it is bound to albumin) by becoming attached to intracellular proteins in the liver; it is then excreted in the bile. The rate of reduction in serum concentration of BSP is a sensitive measure of hepatocellular function.

Indication

The test may be used to assess hepatocellular function, particularly in the absence of jaundice; it may also be used for following the progress of hepatitis. Jaundice, however, is not a contraindication, but biliary obstruction can interfere with interpretation of the test.

Patient Preparation

No special preparation is required.

Protocol

BSP (5 mg/kg body weight) is administered intravenously as a 5% w/v aqueous solution (i.e. a concentration of 5 g/100 ml) over a period of 30 seconds, care being taken that the solution is crystal-free. A venous blood sample (5 ml) is taken into a plain glass bottle at 1 min, and further samples are collected 25 and 45 min following the injection. **Caution: care must be taken to avoid performing the test in those subjects sensitive to BSP, and also to avoid leakage of BSP around the injection site.**

Sample Handling

Serum samples are estimated for BSP.

Normal Response

The 1 min serum sample should show a BSP concentration of 10 mg/100 ml with <15% remaining at 25 min and <7% at 45 min.

Interpretation

Haemorrhage, shock, heart failure, trauma, surgery, fever, and impaired portal circulation interfere with the test. Impaired excre-

13

tion, particularly at 45 min, in the absence of disordered circulation and biliary obstruction, indicates impaired hepatocellular function (including that caused by drugs). Hypoalbuminaemia delays clearance, but albuminuria increases it. Up to 50% BSP retention is seen at 45 min in advanced cirrhosis of the liver. Oestrogen therapy delays BSP excretion by the liver. A falsely low figure for the 45 min serum sample may be caused by an inadequate injection, but under these circumstances the 1 min sample will also be low, failing to attain a level of 10 mg/100 ml. Elderly subjects show slight impairment of excretion. In the Dubin-Johnson syndrome, a 2 h sample contains a higher serum concentration (i.e. there is a secondary rise) than the usual value found at 45 min, although this is not diagnostic of the condition, because the same may occur in other hepatobiliary disorders. In the Rotor type of hyperbilirubinaemia, there is no secondary rise of BSP, but there is increased retention of about 35% at 45 min. In liver storage diseases, there is impaired hepatic uptake and storage of BSP to a more marked degree than in the Rotor syndrome. The patient should be warned that the urine, when alkaline, will appear red following this test.

Comment

This test is now rarely used as a means of assessing hepatocellular function.

BUTTER FAT ABSORPTION TEST

Principle

Following an oral load of butter, the appearance of turbidity due to chylomicrons, in previously clear serum, quantifies the degree of fat absorption.

Indication

This test is useful as a preliminary investigation for excluding general malabsorption, in order to avoid unnecessary performance of fat balance studies.

Patient Preparation

The patient fasts overnight for a period of 14 h and rests in bed for the duration of the investigation. Smoking is not permitted.

Protocol

Venous blood (5 ml) is collected into a plain glass bottle. Orange juice, toast and 500 mg/kg body weight of butter are given orally, followed (if desired) by unsweetened tea or coffee, without milk. A further blood sample (5 ml) is taken at 2 h.

Sample Handling

The blood samples are dispatched routinely to the laboratory for measurement of chylomicrons in the serum.

Normal Response

There is an increase of >20 LSI (light scattering intensity) units in serum at 2 h when compared with the fasting level.

Interpretation

A rise of >20 LSI units in serum at 2 h normally excludes the necessity for carrying out fat balance studies, unless clinical suspicion of malabsorption is very high.

Comment

This is a simple, but useful, screening test.

CALCIUM DEPRIVATION (SODIUM PHYTATE) TEST

Principle

Sodium phytate chelates calcium. When added to a diet already low in calcium, phytate reduces availability of the remaining calcium for absorption to a minimum. This leads to maximal stimulation of the parathyroid glands, which would normally maintain the serum calcium within the reference range by secreting parathyroid hormone (PTH); failure to do so indicates early hypoparathyroidism.

Indication

This test is indicated in patients at risk from hypoparathyroidism, particularly following thyroidectomy, in whom marginal damage to the parathyroid glands is suspected.

Patient Preparation

The patient is placed on a low calcium diet (<300 mg/day), commencing 3 days before the test. Sodium phytate (9 g) is then given orally each day in divided doses with meals for 7 days.

Protocol

Venous blood (5 ml) is taken, following an overnight fast, for estimation of serum calcium and albumin prior to commencing the test, twice during administration of the sodium phytate, and again at the end of the test period. Care must be taken to avoid venous stasis.

Sample Handling

This is as for estimation of serum calcium and albumin.

Normal Response

The serum calcium remains within the reference range when corrected for albumin.

Interpretation

Patients with suspected early hypoparathyroidism may show a

16

base-line serum calcium towards the lower limit of the reference range. If, following administration of sodium phytate, this falls to definitely below the lower limit, the diagnosis of hypoparathyroidism is strengthened.

Comment

In congenital hypoparathyroidism, the biochemical features of low serum calcium and high serum phosphate, with allowance being made for age in children, are usually gross, and this test is not indicated. It is in acquired hypoparathyroidism that marginal changes may be present, and this is the situation in which the test is most useful.

CALCIUM INFUSION TEST
For calcitonin (CT) release

Principle

Calcium infusion causes rapid calcitonin (CT) release from certain tumours, especially medullary carcinoma of the thyroid gland (MCT).

Indication

This test is of value in assessing cases of suspected MCT and other CT-secreting tumours, including some neoplasms of the breast and lung. It may be used to monitor therapeutic response and to detect recurrence of tumour at an early stage following surgical removal.

Patient Preparation

The patient fasts overnight and during the test, remaining at rest in bed. Smoking is not permitted.

Protocol

An intravenous infusion of calcium gluconate (available as a 10% solution, i.e. a concentration of 1 g calcium gluconate/10 ml solution) in 500 ml of physiological saline (5 mg calcium/kg body weight/h) is set up over a period of 3 h (calcium gluconate 11.2 g is approximately equivalent to 1 g calcium). Venous blood (5 ml) is collected at 0, 3 and 4 h into polythene bottles containing heparin, pre-cooled on ice for plasma CT estimation (special collection, see Appendix III). **Caution: hypercalcaemia should be excluded before commencing this test.**

Sample Handling

This is as for plasma CT estimation; samples should be processed immediately. Visible haemolysis invalidates the results.

Normal Response

The plasma CT rises to a peak level of <265 ng/L in males and to <120 ng/L in females from the reference range of <100 ng/L in males and <50 ng/L in females.

Interpretation

Base-line plasma CT levels are normally extremely low; hence, deficiency of CT cannot be readily detected. Raised base-line levels of plasma CT are suggestive of MCT; however, sensitivity is much improved by stimulation with intravenous calcium, which leads to marked elevation if a CT-secreting tumour is present.

Comment

This test has a better detection rate than the shorter calcium infusion tests, but is more time-consuming and gives rise to more side effects in patients with tumours. Side effects include flushing and diarrhoea. Intravenous calcium is only one of several factors known to increase CT release; others include pentagastrin and whisky.

CALCIUM INFUSION TEST
For gastrin release

Principle

Calcium infusion causes gastrin release from gastrin-producing cells. In patients with the Zollinger-Ellison syndrome there is an exaggerated response.

Indication

This test is indicated in patients with suspected Zollinger–Ellison syndrome due to gastrinoma, either in the pancreas (alone or as part of the pluriglandular syndrome) or elsewhere (e.g. gastric antrum, duodenum), or antral G-cell hyperplasia.

Patient Preparation

The patient fasts overnight and during the test and remains at rest in bed. Smoking is not permitted.

Protocol

An intravenous infusion of calcium gluconate (available as a 10% solution, i.e. a concentration of 1 g calcium gluconate/10 ml solution) in 500 ml of physiological saline (5 mg calcium/kg body weight/h) is set up over a period of 3 h (calcium gluconate 11.2 g is approximately equivalent to 1 g calcium). Venous blood (10 ml) is collected into polythene bottles pre-cooled on ice, each containing heparin and 1 ml of Trasylol, at time 0, and at 30 min intervals thereafter for 4 h, for plasma gastrin estimation (special collection, see Appendix III).

Sample Handling

This is as for plasma gastrin estimation; samples should be processed immediately.

Normal Response

The base-line plasma gastrin in adults should be <100 ng/L (higher in old age), rising only slightly in response to calcium infusion.

Interpretation

In the Zollinger-Ellison syndrome, the base-line plasma gastrin level may be markedly elevated, rising yet further in response to calcium infusion (to >300 ng/L). In those cases where the base-line levels are not markedly raised, a doubling in response to calcium infusion occurs.

Comment

This is a useful test which avoids the necessity for performing gastric intubation. An alternative stimulation procedure for gastrin involves administration of secretin.

CALCIUM TOLERANCE TEST

Principle

In patients with primary or tertiary hyperparathyroidism, failure of the normal inhibition of parathyroid hormone (PTH) release in response to an oral calcium load results in an exaggerated calcaemic response, increased hypercalciuria (calcium intolerance), persisting inappropriately high levels of PTH in serum, and continuing raised urinary excretion of both cyclic AMP (cAMP) and nephrogenous cAMP, with elevated renal clearance of cAMP.

Indication

This test is indicated in patients suspected of suffering from primary or tertiary hyperparathyroidism, especially if normocalcaemic; it is, therefore, applicable in difficult cases of unexplained hypercalciuria.

Patient Preparation

The patient is placed on a low calcium diet of <300 mg/day for 7–10 days prior to the test. During the last 2 days of this period, two 24 h urine collections are made for measurement of base-line creatinine, calcium, cAMP and nephrogenous cAMP; in addition, 2 venous blood samples (10 ml) are taken, each following an overnight fast, for serum creatinine, calcium, PTH and cAMP determinations. Prior to commencing the procedure, the patient again fasts overnight, and also during the first 4 h of the test, remaining at rest in bed. Smoking is not permitted.

Protocol

The patient is given 500 ml of water to drink in order to ensure adequate urine output. Elemental calcium (1000 mg) in the form of calcium gluconate is administered orally over a few minutes in a further 200 ml of water (calcium gluconate 11.2 g is approximately equivalent to 1 g calcium). Venous blood (10 ml) is taken at 2 and 4 h for estimation of serum creatinine, calcium, albumin, PTH (special collection, see Appendix III) and cAMP. Over the next 24 h all urine is collected in 4 h samples for assay of creatinine, calcium, cAMP and nephrogenous cAMP.

22

Sample Handling

Samples are handled as for serum creatinine, calcium, albumin, PTH and cAMP estimation. Urine volumes are measured and samples are handled as for urinary creatinine, calcium and cAMP.

Normal Response

Normal subjects exhibit only a slight rise in serum calcium (corrected for albumin) and urinary calcium excretion, but usually within the reference ranges; complete suppression of serum PTH, and moderate suppression of urinary excretion and clearance of cAMP and excretion of nephrogenous cAMP should also occur.

Interpretation

Patients with primary or tertiary hyperparathyroidism respond to a calcium load by exhibiting a marked rise in serum calcium (whether originally normocalcaemic or hypercalcaemic) and a marked increase in the already high urine calcium excretion, thus indicating intolerance to calcium. Of greater importance, however, is the failure of suppression of PTH production and of both cAMP clearance and nephrogenous cAMP excretion. Patients with absorptive hypercalciuria also show a calcaemic response, but, in addition, there is marked suppression of nephrogenous cAMP excretion. Patients with renal tubular hypercalciuria show a small calcaemic response and minimal reduction in nephrogenous cAMP excretion.

Comment

This is an important test, only occasionally required, but may be particularly relevant when reliable serum PTH assays are not readily available. Calcium loading is not without danger in the presence of significant hypercalcaemia.

CALORIE RESTRICTION TEST

Principle

Calorie restriction stresses the impaired hepatocyte transport defect for unconjugated bilirubin in Gilbert's syndrome, in which there is intracellular endoplasmic UDP glucuronyl transferase deficiency. As a result there is an excessive rise in both serum unconjugated and total bilirubin.

Indication

This test is indicated in patients with suspected Gilbert's syndrome, particularly those presenting after infective hepatitis with persistent hyperbilirubinaemia as a lone feature.

Patient Preparation

The patient should have been taking a normal diet for at least one week and should not be receiving enzyme-inducing medication, particularly phenobarbitone. Smoking is not permitted throughout the test period.

Protocol

A base-line venous blood sample (5 ml) is taken for estimation of serum unconjugated and total bilirubin. Following this, the patient is placed on a 400 calorie intake for 24 h, e.g. Slender (The Boots Company plc) prepared with water (not milk), at the end of which a repeat venous blood sample (5 ml) is collected.

Sample Handling

This is as for estimation of serum bilirubin. The samples should be protected from light and dispatched immediately to the laboratory.

Normal Response

There is a small rise in serum total bilirubin (but to not $>25 \mu$mol/L), most of which is unconjugated.

Interpretation

Patients with Gilbert's syndrome have as a lone biochemical feature a raised base-line serum total bilirubin level, but $<50 \mu$mol/L, most

24

of which is unconjugated; the level may double in response to this procedure.

Comment

This is a simple and reliable test but is required only in cases of genuine diagnostic doubt.

CHLORPROMAZINE STIMULATION TEST

Principle

Chlorpromazine, being a phenothiazine compound, acts as a dopamine-blocking agent. It causes secretion of prolactin (PRL) from the anterior pituitary gland, by removing the normal inhibitory action of dopamine produced in the hypothalamus. Measurement of the serum PRL response allows assessment of hypothalamic function.

Indication

This test is indicated in suspected hypothalamic disease.

Patient Preparation

The patient fasts overnight and during the test and should remain at rest in bed. Smoking is not permitted. Anxiety must be alleviated. An intravenous catheter is inserted into the antecubital vein at least 30 min prior to commencing the test. Dopamine-blocking drugs (such as phenothiazines), and dopamine-depleting drugs (such as α-methyldopa) must be avoided for several days previously.

Protocol

Chlorpromazine (25 mg for adults; 0.4 mg/kg body weight for children) is injected intramuscularly. Venous blood (5 ml) is collected at 0, 60, 90, 120 and 180 min into plain glass bottles.

Sample Handling

This is as for serum PRL estimation.

Normal Response

There should be at least a 3-fold increase in serum PRL during the test period.

Interpretation

Failure of the 3-fold rise from a normal base-line level is indicative of hypothalamic damage. No such interpretation can be made if the base-line level is already elevated as a result of stress, other drugs or a PRL-secreting tumour, i.e. prolactinoma (which may be a micro-tumour).

Comment

This is a rarely used test. The side effects which may occur are those related to chlorpromazine administration.

CLOMIPHENE STIMULATION TEST

Principle

Clomiphene citrate is a non-steroidal compound which blocks hypothalamic steroid receptors, thereby preventing natural gonadal steroids from producing a negative feedback to the hypothalamus. There is, as a result, release of gonadotrophin-releasing hormone (Gn-RH, luteinizing hormone/follicle-stimulating hormone-releasing hormone, LH/FSH-RH) which causes increased secretion of luteinizing hormone (LH) and follicle-stimulating hormone (FSH) from the anterior pituitary gland.

Indication

This test is indicated for differentiating delayed puberty from isolated hypogonadotrophic hypogonadism. It may also be used in conjunction with the 'Gonadotrophin-releasing hormone (Gn-RH, luteinizing hormone/follicle-stimulating hormone-releasing hormone, LH/FSH-RH) stimulation test', for differentiating hypothalamic from pituitary lesions.

Patient Preparation

No special preparation is required, but the patient should not have been receiving steroid compounds. The test may be performed on in-patients or out-patients.

Protocol

For adult males, clomiphene citrate (100 mg) is administered twice daily by mouth for 11 days. Adult females should receive clomiphene citrate (100 mg) daily by mouth for 5 days, commencing on the 5th day of the menstrual cycle. Venous blood (10 ml) should be collected into a plain glass bottle before commencing the drug and again on each of the last 3 days.

Sample Handling

This is as for estimation of serum testosterone, FSH and LH.

Normal Response

In adult males, serum testosterone and FSH should rise by >50%

27

and serum LH by >75% from base-line levels within the reference range. In adult females, serum LH and FSH should at least double, rising from base-line levels within the reference range.

Interpretation

In response to this test, elevation of serum LH occurs, not only in normal subjects, but also in patients with primary testicular disease, the latter exhibiting a high base-line level of serum LH with reduced serum testosterone. Males before puberty, patients with hypothalamic or pituitary disease and those with isolated LH deficiency show reduced or absent responses of serum LH, FSH and testosterone from low base-line levels.

Comment

This test is only rarely carried out in practice, but it does add to the value of the measurement of base-line serum LH levels in aiding differentiation of primary from secondary hypogonadism in the male. In the female, complications in the form of over-stimulation of the ovaries may result in cystic ovarian changes and multiple pregnancies, particularly if the test is prolonged for more than 5 days.

28

CLONIDINE STIMULATION TEST

Principle

Clonidine stimulates growth hormone (GH) release from the anterior pituitary gland. Following administration, clonidine causes elevation of serum GH levels, measurements of which serve as a test of anterior pituitary function.

Indication

This test is indicated in suspected GH deficiency.

Patient Preparation

The patient should be investigated under 'basal conditions'(see Appendix I), except that there is no restriction on water intake.

Protocol

Clonidine is administered orally as 25 μg Dixarit tablets (Boehringer Ingelheim Ltd) in a dose of 0.15 mg/m^2 of body surface area, and rounded up to the nearest whole number of tablets. Blood pressure is monitored at 30 min intervals throughout the test and for a further 3 h afterwards. Venous blood (5 ml) is collected at 0, 30, 60, 90, 120, 150 and 180 min into plain glass bottles. An intravenous catheter, inserted 30 min prior to collection of the first blood sample, should be used. **Caution: drowsiness and hypotension may be side effects for up to 3 h, and continuing bed rest is, therefore, essential.**

Sample Handling

This is as for serum GH estimation.

Normal Response

There is a steep rise of serum GH from <10 mIU/L initially to >20 mIU/L at 60–120 min after clonidine administration.

Interpretation

An inadequate response is seen in GH deficiency, either as an isolated state, or as part of panhypopituitarism; a poor response may also occur in primary hypothyroidism. In some children, social deprivation also leads to inadequate response.

Comment

This test is safer than insulin-induced hypoglycaemia, especially in children; however, it tests only GH release, as compared with the latter test which stimulates the whole of the hypothalamo-pituitary-adrenal axis. Clonidine is a stronger stimulus for GH release than L-arginine, Bovril, L-dopa, glucagon or insulin.

CORTICOTROPHIN-RELEASING FACTOR (CRF) STIMULATION TEST

Principle

Corticotrophin-releasing factor (CRF) is a synthetic preparation of the 41 amino acid residue peptide isolated from ovine hypothalami. When administered to man, CRF specifically causes elevation of plasma ACTH and serum cortisol, thus serving as a clinical test of pituitary ACTH reserve.

Indication

This test may be used either alone or in combination with other hypothalamic-releasing hormone stimulation tests. It differentiates between hypothalamic and pituitary disorders of ACTH secretion.

Patient Preparation

The patient should be investigated under 'basal conditions'(see Appendix I), except that there is no restriction on water intake.

Protocol

Venous blood (5 ml) is collected into glass bottles containing heparin for estimation of plasma ACTH (special collection, see Appendix III) and into plain glass bottles prior to the intravenous injection of 100 μg CRF (Bachem UK Ltd) in 1 ml acid saline (pH 2.0) over a period of 1 min. Further blood samples are collected at 20 and 60 min. An intravenous catheter is inserted at least 30 min prior to blood sampling.

Sample Handling

This is as for plasma ACTH and serum cortisol estimation.

Normal Response

The plasma ACTH should rise from levels within the reference range by at least 50% in either the 30 or 60 min sample. The serum cortisol should rise from within the reference range by at least 50% in the 60 min sample.

31

Interpretation

In patients with pituitary-dependent Cushing's disease, CRF stimulation causes the plasma ACTH to rise excessively from an already elevated base-line level; the serum cortisol level also displays a rise, the hyper-responsiveness being of much longer duration than in the normal individual. In adrenocortical over-activity, associated with high serum cortisol, there is low or undetectable plasma ACTH both before and after a CRF injection and there is no cortisol response. In patients with an ectopic ACTH-producing tumour, there is characteristically no increase of either plasma ACTH or serum cortisol in this test. In patients with hypopituitarism secondary to hypothalamic disease, there is a marked rise in plasma ACTH from a low base-line level after CRF administration, but there is no increase in serum cortisol at 60 min. In isolated ACTH deficiency there is no change in ACTH after CRF, both plasma ACTH and serum cortisol remaining below the lower limit of detection. In patients with isolated adrenocortical insufficiency, including Addison's disease, CRF stimulation causes a significant rise in plasma ACTH from an already raised base-line level, whereas the serum cortisol level does not change.

Comment

This is a recently introduced test which awaits full evaluation in the clinical context. Delayed responses in hypothalamic disorders have not yet been described. This test may form part of a series of pituitary investigations, as the response is highly specific. The side effect of transient facial warmth is minimal.

CREATININE CLEARANCE TEST

Principle

Creatinine clearance is the theoretical volume of blood which is wholly cleared of creatinine following one passage through the kidney. It is a measure of glomerular function, based on the assumption that there is neither excretion nor absorption of creatinine by the renal tubules.

Indication

This test is used for assessing renal glomerular function (glomerular filtration rate, GFR) for both diagnostic and management purposes in chronic renal disease. It is also used serially to measure the progress of renal disease, and to detect kidney rejection at an early stage following transplantation.

Patient Preparation

No special preparation is required, other than to encourage the patient to drink freely the night before. This is in order to produce a sufficient and constant urine flow, so that accurate urine collection can be made, especially when 2 periods of 1 h urine collections are made, as opposed to the 24 h collection, i.e. to establish a flow of approximately 1–2 ml/min.

Protocol

Measurements of height and weight are made to permit calculation of body surface area in the case of children. For the 1 h 'Creatinine clearance test' the bladder is emptied and the urine discarded. An approximately 1 h sample of urine is collected; the timing should be accurate and precise to within 1 min. Venous blood (5 ml) is collected into a plain glass bottle approximately half-way through the 1 h urine collection. A second 1 h urine collection is made immediately following the first, together with a second blood sample. The bladder must be emptied completely, both at the beginning and end of each 1 h period, preferably with supra-pubic pressure. The urine samples are collected into 2 plain glass bottles, each of 250 ml capacity, without preservative. For the 24 h 'Creatinine clearance test', a 24 h urine sample is collected accurately; venous blood (5 ml) is also collected into a plain glass bottle during this period.

33

Sample Handling

This is as for serum and urine creatinine estimation. The urine volumes are measured.

Normal Response

The normal creatinine clearance is 100–120 ml/min.

Interpretation

Creatinine clearance values of <90 ml/min indicate renal impairment. In advanced disease, clearances of <10 ml/min are encountered. However, 70% of kidney destruction is necessary before significant impairment of creatinine clearance becomes evident. There is a tendency for creatinine clearance to fall in the elderly. The test is independent of dietary protein intake and endogenous protein breakdown, differing in this respect from the now rarely used test of urea clearance. In paediatric practice, body surface area correction is necessary; clearance should, therefore, be expressed as ml/min/1.73 m^2.

Comment

The 1 h 'Creatinine clearance test', carried out with close duplicate results, provides a more accurate assessment than the 24 h 'Creatinine clearance test', assuming the protocol is followed closely, particularly with respect to the accurate timing of urine collections. Carefully monitored serum creatinine alone is now more frequently used to assess renal function serially, particularly following renal transplantation. However, determination of creatinine clearance remains a simple, useful, reliable and inexpensive test of renal function. The test described here measures endogenous creatinine clearance; exogenous creatinine clearance estimation, in which an oral load of creatinine is given to the patient, is not now in routine use. The 'Inulin clearance test', although more accurate, is a rarely used test of glomerular function.

DESFERRIOXAMINE CHELATION TEST

Principle

Desferrioxamine mesylate competes with transferrin for iron *in vivo*. It chelates iron, forming a water-soluble complex, which is readily excreted by the kidney. Measurement of iron in the urine during this test, therefore, forms the basis for assessing the body stores of iron.

Indication

This test is useful for the demonstration of increased tissue iron stores, particularly in idiopathic haemochromatosis. It may be used, in association with repeated venesection, to monitor iron depletion therapy in this condition. It may also be indicated for the relatives of a patient with known haemochromatosis.

Patient Preparation

The patient should receive vitamin C (10 mg/kg body weight) daily for 7 days prior to the test to standardise the excretion of iron.

Protocol

Desferrioxamine mesylate (500 mg) is administered intramuscularly and 400 ml water is taken orally to ensure adequate urine output. At the same time, the bladder is emptied and the urine discarded. All urine is then collected in an acid-washed iron-free polythene bottle over the next 6 h for iron estimation (special collection, see Appendix III).

Sample Handling

This is as for estimation of iron in urine.

Normal Response

In the normal subject 18–27 μmol of iron is excreted in the 6 h period.

Interpretation

Increased excretion of iron occurs in all states of tissue iron overload, including idiopathic haemochromatosis, transfusion haemosiderosis, the siderosis seen in the South African Bantu, and where there is an elevated iron content in the liver associated with cirrhosis. Results are most meaningful clinically when there is very high excretion of iron, as in haemochromatosis. Results are valid only if renal function is normal.

Comment

A modification of this test involves measurement of radioactive iron in the urine following oral administration of ^{59}Fe. Diethylene-triamine penta-acetic acid (DTPA) is sometimes used as an alternative chelating agent, although interpretation of the excretion patterns is different.

DESMOPRESSIN ACETATE
(1-Deamino-8-D-arginine vasopressin, DDAVP) RESPONSE TEST

Principle

Exogenously administered desmopressin acetate (1-deamino-8-D-arginine vasopressin, DDAVP) fails to lessen the diuresis in either congenital or acquired nephrogenic diabetes insipidus. These disorders are characterised by renal tubular end-organ resistance to vasopressin, thus differentiating them from hypothalamic/pituitary diabetes insipidus, in which conditions a positive response occurs in this test.

Indication

The test is used to confirm the diagnosis of nephrogenic diabetes insipidus.

Patient Preparation

For several hours prior to the test, free access to fluids is encouraged. Smoking is not permitted. **Caution: this test could precipitate water intoxication in association with marked but temporary urine suppression.**

Protocol

In the morning, the bladder is emptied completely, the urine being saved in a plain glass bottle. Venous blood (5 ml) is collected into a plain glass bottle. The aqueous preparation of DDAVP ($4 \mu g$) is then administered intramuscularly, and further samples of venous blood and urine are collected at hourly intervals for a period of 4 h.

Sample Handling

This is as for estimation of sodium, potassium and osmolality in serum, and osmolality in urine. Urine volumes are also recorded.

Normal Response

There should be a marked fall in urine volume and a marked rise in osmolality. The serum osmolality should be reduced to near the lower limit of the reference range (280 mmol/kg) and, although the serum sodium concentration may also fall slightly, it should, nevertheless, remain within the reference range, as also should serum potassium.

Interpretation

Patients with nephrogenic diabetes insipidus will fail to respond adequately to DDAVP, maintaining a high urine output of low osmolality, with serum osmolality above the upper limit of the reference range (290 mmol/kg). The serum sodium concentration will be near to or above the upper limit of the reference range. Patients with pituitary or hypothalamic diabetes insipidus or psychogenic polydipsia respond to DDAVP administration by showing a fall in urine volume and a rise in osmolality, though in the latter disorder the response may take several days to become fully manifested. Indeed, patients with a marked and prolonged diuresis from any cause may respond poorly to DDAVP initially.

Comment

It is not appropriate to perform this test in patients with polyuria due to chronic renal failure or osmotic diuresis. Serum potassium measurements are indicated when there is prolonged urinary suppression following DDAVP, though this is less likely to occur than was the case with the earlier long-acting oily preparations of vasopressin. Interpretation of this test should be considered in conjuction with the 'Water deprivation test'.

DEXAMETHASONE SUPPRESSION TEST (DST)
Multiple high dose

Principle
A high dose of dexamethasone, administered over a short period of time, differentiates pituitary-dependent Cushing's disease from Cushing's syndrome of other aetiology by causing suppression of plasma ACTH and serum cortisol in the former.

Indication
This test is useful in helping to determine the cause of established Cushing's syndrome and particularly in the differentiation of pituitary-dependent Cushing's disease from the other causes of Cushing's syndrome, including ectopic ACTH-production by tumours, adrenocortical adenomas and adrenocortical carcinomas; the latter 3 disorders do not usually show suppression.

Patient Preparation
The patient should be admitted to hospital. There should have been no treatment with glucocorticoid drugs (including topical preparations) for several weeks; mineralocorticoids do not interfere with this test. The test should not be performed in the presence of cardiac failure.

Protocol
Dexamethasone (2 mg) is administered orally every 6 h over a period of 48 h, i.e. a total of 16 mg is given. Venous blood (5 ml) is collected into a plain glass bottle for serum cortisol and 20 ml into a polythene bottle containing heparin pre-cooled on ice for plasma ACTH estimation (special collection, see Appendix III), immediately before starting the test and again 6 h after the last dose of dexamethasone.

Sample Handling
This is as for estimation of serum cortisol and plasma ACTH; the sample for ACTH estimation should be processed immediately.

Normal Response
There is marked suppression of serum cortisol to <50% of the

39

base-line level 6 h after the last dose of dexamethasone.

Interpretation

Suppression of serum cortisol to <50% of the base-line level in patients with Cushing's syndrome points to a pituitary-dependent aetiology. This response also occurs in alcohol-induced Cushing's syndrome. Failure of suppression to this degree is a feature of both adrenocortical tumours (adenoma and carcinoma) and ectopic ACTH-producing tumours. Misleading results, with both suppression and failure of suppression, can occur; failure of suppression occurs particularly in some patients with pituitary disease. Measurement of base-line plasma ACTH discriminates between adrenocortical tumours in which it is low, and ectopic ACTH-producing tumours in which it is high. An extremely high serum cortisol level favours the diagnosis of adrenocortical carcinoma or ectopic ACTH-producing tumour. A 'paradoxical response' (i.e. a rise of serum cortisol) to dexamethasone administration should alert one to the possibility of cyclical Cushing's syndrome.

Comment

This test is time-consuming and not without adverse clinical effects, particularly in patients with incipient cardiac failure, hypertension and peptic ulcer. It is currently less frequently employed than formerly. Suppression of a high base-line plasma ACTH following dexamethasone administration occurs in patients with pituitary-dependent Cushing's disease, but adds nothing to the information gained from confirming cortisol suppression alone. Dexamethasone does not interfere with the measurement of serum cortisol.

DEXAMETHASONE SUPPRESSION TEST (DST)
Single low dose for Cushing's syndrome

Principle

In Cushing's syndrome due to any cause, a standard low dose (2 mg) of dexamethasone fails to suppress the serum cortisol. Suppression of cortisol excludes clinically suspected Cushing's syndrome.

Indication

This test is indicated for excluding Cushing's syndrome suspected on clinical grounds or biochemical grounds, i.e. patients with a high serum cortisol with loss of circadian rhythm.

Patient Preparation

There should have been no treatment with glucocorticoid drugs (including topical preparations) for several weeks; mineralocorticoids do not interfere with this test. The test may be performed on in-patients or out-patients.

Protocol

Venous blood (5 ml) is collected into a plain glass bottle at 8.00–9.00 am. Dexamethasone (2 mg) is given orally at 11.00 pm on the same day and a further blood sample is taken at 9.00 am the following morning.

Sample Handling

This is as for estimation of serum cortisol.

Normal Response

There is marked suppression of serum cortisol to <180 nmol/L at 8.00–9.00 am on the second morning, and/or a fall of >50% of the base-line level, the reference range for serum cortisol at 9.00 am being 140–640 nmol/L.

Interpretation

Adequate suppression of cortisol as revealed by the serum level at 8.00–9.00 am on the second day, makes the diagnosis of Cushing's syndrome very unlikely. Failure of suppression does not necessarily

41

confirm the diagnosis of Cushing's syndrome, nor does it differentiate the different causes which include pituitary adenomas with adrenocortical hyperplasia, adrenocortical tumours, ectopic ACTH-producing tumours, and alcoholism; it should be noted that the raised serum cortisol levels found in obesity and endogenous depression are also not suppressed in this test. Where there is a 'paradoxical response' (i.e. a rise in serum cortisol) to dexamethasone administration, the possibility of cyclical Cushing's syndrome should be considered.

Comment

This is a screening procedure which may be followed by the multiple high dose 'Dexamethasone suppression test (DST)'. Marked hepatic microsomal P450 enzyme induction, as caused by a number of drugs (e.g. phenobarbitone, other anticonvulsants and benzodiazepines) may interfere with the test by causing dexamethasone to be eliminated unduly rapidly, thereby causing inadequate suppression of serum cortisol (see page 44). It should be noted that in cases of virilising tumours in females, suppression of serum testosterone in this test more often occurs when the source is adrenal, although dexamethasone can sometimes suppress the production of testosterone by ovarian tumours. Dexamethasone does not interfere with the measurement of serum cortisol.

DEXAMETHASONE SUPPRESSION TEST (DST)[4]
Single low dose for depression

Principle

The normal response of serum cortisol suppression, following a standard dose of dexamethasone given orally, is absent in approximately 50% of patients suffering from affective disorders with a significant element of endogenous depression, due to failure of negative feed-back to suppress the limbic system.

Indication

This test is indicated in patients with affective disorders in whom there is clinical suspicion of endogenous depression.

Patient Preparation

There should have been no treatment with glucocorticoid drugs (including topical preparations) for several weeks; mineralocorticoids do not interfere with this test. The test may be performed on in-patients or out-patients.

Protocol

Venous blood (5 ml) is taken into a plain glass bottle at 9.00 am and 4.00 pm on the first day. At 11.00 pm on the same evening, dexamethasone (1 mg) is given orally. A further blood sample is taken at 9.00 am and 4.00 pm on the following day.

Sample Handling

This is as for serum cortisol estimation.

Normal Response

The base-line 9.00 am serum cortisol value on the first day should be within the reference range (140–640 nmol/L). There is marked suppression of the 9.00 am serum cortisol value on the second day (i.e. 10 h after the dexamethasone dose); this remains low at 4.00 pm (<180 nmol/L), persisting for a total period of 24 h.

Interpretation

A significant proportion of patients with depression (in whom there

43

is loss of the normal diurnal variation in serum cortisol levels) show early 'escape' from the suppression of serum cortisol normally seen at 4.00 pm on the second day, as evidenced by a concentration of >180 nmol/L, or of >50% of the value found at 4.00 pm on the first day; however, many patients with depression fail to show this 'escape' by exhibiting a low serum cortisol concentration at this time, i.e. a false negative result. Low serum cortisol concentrations may also be found in individuals with organic hypofunction of the adrenal cortex or anterior pituitary gland, but these patients would show low levels in the base-line sample, too. Marked hepatic micro-somal P450 enzyme induction by drugs leads to dexamethasone being eliminated rapidly, thereby causing inadequate suppression of serum cortisol (see page 42). Some patients with other disorders, including anorexia nervosa without obvious depression, weight loss from other causes and patients with dementia associated with enlarged cerebral ventricles, show false positive responses, i.e. they, too, display 'escape' from suppression; 20% of normal subjects also show a positive response. The test is negative in patients with pure anxiety states and schizophrenia, but it must be remembered that these disorders may be associated with an element of depression, in which case the test could be positive. A repeat test, following treatment for the depression, which remains positive, suggests a poor prognosis.

Comment

If the 9.00 am blood sample taken on the second day shows a low serum cortisol concentration, as compared with a normal base-line value on the first day, this confirms compliance with the taking of an adequate dose of dexamethasone. This knowledge is important when assessing depressed patients exhibiting early 'escape', i.e. by finding normal serum cortisol levels at 4.00 pm on the second day. Some authorities recommend measurement of serum dexametha-sone concentrations as a further check on compliance, in addition to assaying serum cortisol. Dexamethasone does not interfere with the measurement of serum cortisol. There is wide discussion and some difference of opinion in the literature concerning the value of this test, and some authorities would advocate a prolonged suppres-sion test, in which there would be increased significance of a positive result.

L-DOPA STIMULATION TEST

Principle

L-Dopa stimulates growth hormone (GH) secretion from the anterior pituitary gland. Following administration, L-dopa causes elevation of serum GH levels, measurements of which serve as a test of anterior pituitary function.

Indication

This test is used in patients suspected of having GH deficiency.

Preparation

The patient should be investigated under 'basal conditions' (see Appendix I), except that there is no restriction on water intake.

Protocol

L-Dopa (500 mg) is administered orally in the case of adults; the dose for children weighing less than 15 kg is 125 mg, but for those of 15–30 kg the dose is 250 mg. Venous blood (5 ml) is collected at 0, 20, 40, 60, 90 and 120 min after the oral L-dopa administration into plain glass bottles. An intravenous catheter, inserted 30 min prior to collection of the first blood sample, should be used.

Sample Handling

This is as for serum GH estimation

Normal Response

Serum GH levels, commencing at <10 mIU/L, should rise to >20 mIU/L or show an increment of >10 mIU/L; peak values occur at 60–120 min.

Interpretation

A normal response excludes GH deficiency, either as part of panhypopituitarism or as an isolated defect. Impaired responses may occur in primary hypothyroidism and 15% of normal subjects.

L-Dopa stimulation test

Comment

In view of the impaired response seen in some normal subjects, the test is of greater value in excluding GH deficiency by the finding of normal values, than in serving as a confirmatory test of such deficiency. An impaired response should be confirmed by other GH-stimulatory tests. This test is the best alternative to the 'Insulin stress test' for hypothalamic-pituitary (anterior) assessment in adults, but other stimulants are available; these include L-arginine, Bovril, clonidine, glucagon, and insulin. Side effects of this test may include transient nausea and occasional vomiting.

ELSWORTH-HOWARD TEST (MODIFIED)

Principle

Parathyroid hormone (PTH) of demonstrated potency, when administered to patients with hypoparathyroidism, differentiates primary hypoparathyroidism from pseudohypoparathyroidism. The basis is that patients with the latter condition, in which there is tissue end-organ resistance to the hormone, do not respond by exhibiting the normal increased urinary excretion of cyclic AMP (cAMP).

Indication

This test is indicated in patients with suspected pseudohypoparathyroidism.

Patient Preparation

The patient should fast overnight and during the test, but should be encouraged to drink water freely, in order to ensure an adequate urine output; caffeine-containing drinks are prohibited. Smoking is not permitted.

Protocol

Measurements of height and weight are made for the purpose of calculating body surface area. Synthetic human PTH (1–34) (300 USP units/1.73 m^2 body surface area) in 50 ml 0.9% sodium chloride is infused intravenously over 15 min. Venous blood (10 ml) is collected into a plain polythene bottle for serum PTH determination (special collection, see Appendix III) prior to the injection of synthetic PTH. A 1 h urine sample is also collected into a plain glass bottle prior to the injection, followed by 2 samples of 30 min each and a further sample of 1 h immediately following the injection, all for cAMP estimation.

Specimen Handling

This is as for serum PTH and urinary cAMP estimation, measurements also being made of the volumes of all separate urine specimens.

47

Normal Response

The base-line serum PTH is within the reference range. There should be a >10-fold increase in urinary cAMP excretion in this test.

Interpretation

In pseudohypoparathyroidism the base-line serum PTH level will be raised. In post-surgical or idiopathic hypoparathyroidism, serum PTH will be depressed or non-detectable. The urinary cAMP excretion in pseudohypoparathyroidism will rise by only 3- to 4-fold in response to the PTH injection, but in primary hypoparathyroidism it rises by >50-fold. Where there is an impaired response, biological activity of the injected PTH should be confirmed in a normal control.

Comment

This protocol is more reliable than earlier ones involving a phosphaturic response to bovine PTH, and differentiates pseudohypoparathyroidism clearly from the other groups.

ETHYLENEDIAMINE TETRA-ACETIC ACID (EDTA) CHELATION TEST

Principle

The calcium disodium salt of ethylenediamine tetra-acetic acid (EDTA) chelates lead from bone, red cells and other tissues. The complex in plasma is water-soluble and is readily excreted by the kidneys, thus permitting measurement in urine of the lead removed.

Indication

This test is used in the assessment of both adults and children suspected of having been exposed to lead.

Patient Preparation

No special preparation is required.

Protocol

Calcium disodium EDTA (75 mg/kg body weight, divided into 3 equal doses at 8 h intervals), taken from a 5 ml ampoule containing 1 g of the compound, with 2% procaine (i.e. 40 mg in 2 ml) added in sufficient quantity to make a final procaine concentration of 0.5%, is administered intramuscularly; calcium disodium EDTA is available as Ledclair. Urine samples (24 h) are collected into acid-washed polythene bottles for lead estimation (special collection, see Appendix III). **Caution: rapid chelation of lead from large quantities stored over a long period in bone, may produce high blood levels and cause acute lead intoxication.**

Sample Handling

This is as for estimation of lead in urine.

Normal Response

In both adults and children, the base-line urinary excretion of lead should be $<0.2 \mu$mol/24 h. Following calcium disodium EDTA administration this figure may double.

49

Interpretation

Urinary lead excretion of $>0.4\,\mu$mol/24 h is indicative of exposure to the metal and of potential intoxication. Following calcium disodium EDTA administration figures of up to $>4.0\,\mu$mol/24 h may be found.

Comment

This test should only be used to confirm exposure to lead following estimation, not only of whole blood lead, but also of a base-line urinary excretion of lead. Other tests of lead exposure/intoxication include measurement of δ-aminolaevulinic acid (δ-ALA) dehydratase activity in erythrocyte haemolysates, assessment of urinary δ-ALA excretion, and erythrocyte protoporphyrin determination. Urinary lead excretion is greatly raised following administration of D-penicillamine, used therapeutically in lead intoxication.

FASTING TEST

Principle

Patients with an insulinoma exhibit inappropriately high serum insulin levels due to excessive release from the tumour, resulting in fasting hypoglycaemia. A prolonged fast provides opportunity for the biochemical changes to be fully expressed; exercise, as an additional factor, may be needed to produce symptoms of hypoglycaemia.

Indication

This test is indicated where there is a suspected insulin-secreting tumour, either pancreatic (β-cells of the islets of Langerhans) or extra-pancreatic in origin.

Patient Preparation

No special preparation is required. Prescribed medications should be continued. Smoking is not permitted.

Protocol

The patient commences the fast (say) in the early evening, continuing overnight and for up to 72 h under observation. Free access to 'water only' is allowed throughout this period. Exercise during the daytime, within the capacity of the cardiac and respiratory systems, should be encouraged. Venous blood (5 ml) is collected and divided equally between a glass bottle containing fluoride/oxalate and a plain glass bottle, at least once in the morning and afternoon on each day and also at any other times at which hypoglycaemic symptoms appear. Facilities for resuscitation from marked hypoglycaemia should be available immediately (20 ml of a sterile 50% w/v solution of glucose, i.e. a concentration of 50 g/100 ml water, given intravenously). Should hypoglycaemia occur (confirmed by plasma glucose analysis), then the fast can be terminated; however, it is vital that blood be taken at this important time for serum insulin and C-peptide analysis.

Sample Handling

This is as for plasma glucose, and serum insulin and C-peptide estimations.

51

Normal Response

The plasma glucose should not fall below the lower limit of the fasting reference range (2.5 mmol/L); serum insulin and C-peptide levels should be 'appropriate' for the corresponding plasma glucose values.

Interpretation

The essential criterion for the diagnosis of insulinoma by this test is the demonstration of low plasma glucose levels in absolute terms (with or without clinical features of hypoglycaemia) in association with measurable serum insulin and C-peptide; the presence of both the latter substances is 'inappropriate' in these circumstances. The test is not indicated in suspected reactive hypoglycaemia. Assay of C-peptide is important only if insulin administration is suspected of being a possible cause for the hypoglycaemia, in which case the serum insulin level will be high and the serum C-peptide level low. Surreptitious administration of oral hypoglycaemic drugs raises all serum insulin components, including pro-insulin and C-peptide, in proportion. Pro-insulin is disproportionately raised in the serum of patients with insulinoma, though it is not normally measured.

Comment

This is a simple, important and useful practical test.

FAT BALANCE TEST

Principle

The faecal fat content, measured over a period of 5 days in patients placed on a standard fat intake, is a measure of intestinal fat absorption.

Indication

This test is indicated in patients with suspected steatorrhoea.

Patient Preparation

The patient is placed on a diet containing fat of up to approximately 70 g/day for a period of 5 days. Laxatives should be avoided if possible, but a high fibre content in the diet is helpful in promoting regular daily stool collections. Liquid paraffin is best avoided.

Protocol

A faecal marker dye (e.g. carmine, etc.) is administered orally at the start of the test and the time noted. All stools are collected following the first appearance of the marker. On the fifth day, a second marker is administered orally at the same time of day, all stools continuing to be collected up to its appearance.

Sample Handling

All specimens are collected in cellophane packages, placed into plastic cartons and labelled with the patient's name, the date and the time of collection. The cartons, numbered sequentially, are sent to the laboratory as soon as they are complete.

Normal Response

The average total fatty acid content of the stools collected between the markers over the 5 day period should be <16 mmol/24 h, the stool volume being 100–200 ml/24 h.

Interpretation

A total faecal fatty acid content of >70 mmol/24 h is strong evidence for steatorrhoea of pancreatic origin, perhaps reaching 180 mmol/24 h, with a volume of up to 2 L/24 h. Intestinal malabsorption is typically associated with a lesser excretion of total fatty acids, ranging from 35–70 mmol/24 h. One of the most important causes of intestinal malabsorption is gluten sensitivity; a repeat test on a low gluten diet giving a normal result strongly confirms this diagnosis. Another cause of remediable malabsorption is infestation with the parasite *Giardia lamblia*. Increased faecal fatty acids may also be caused by marked intestinal hurry from any cause.

Comment

This is an unpleasant investigation for the laboratory and should be avoided wherever possible. Many screening tests are available including the 'Butter fat absorption test' and the 'Oleic acid and triolein absorption test'. In gluten sensitivity the definitive investigation is peroral jejunal biopsy. Total faecal fatty acids, expressed in mmol/24 h can be converted to fat in g/24 h by multiplying by 0.284. The degree of fat absorption can be calculated by expressing the daily fat intake minus the daily fat excretion, as a percentage of the daily fat intake, all measurements being made in g/24 h.

9α-FLUDROCORTISONE SUPPRESSION TEST

Principle

9α-Fludrocortisone administration fails to suppress the high plasma aldosterone and high urinary aldosterone excretion in patients with primary hyperaldosteronism (Conn's syndrome).

Indication

This test is used to confirm Conn's syndrome.

Patient Preparation

The patient should take a normal diet and must be under supervision throughout the test. There should have been no diuretic or antihypertensive therapy nor liquorice intake, for 3 weeks prior to the test.

Protocol

9α-Fludrocortisone (0.2 mg) is given orally to adults every 8 h for a total of 9 doses. Two successive 24 h urine samples are collected into polythene bottles, each containing 10 ml of 1% boric acid solution for aldosterone estimation (special collection, see Appendix III), prior to the first dose and all further 24 h samples saved likewise for the next 3 days, with a sixth sample following the last dose of the drug. Venous blood (10 ml) is collected into a polythene bottle containing heparin for plasma aldosterone estimation (special collection, see Appendix III) prior to the first dose of 9α-fludrocortisone, and a further sample 2 h after the last dose, the patient having been lying down for 2 h before each venepuncture.

Sample Handling

Specimens of blood and urine for aldosterone estimation must be sent to the laboratory immediately after collection.

Normal Response

The plasma aldosterone should be <110 pmol/L, and the urine aldosterone <55 nmol/24 h.

Interpretation

Failure to suppress a high base-line aldosterone concentration in the plasma and/or a high excretion in the urine confirms the diagnosis of primary hyperaldosteronism, in which low plasma renin activity would usually already have been demonstrated.

Comment

This is a useful confirmatory test, but is not without danger in patients with severe hypertension, renal impairment, cardiac failure or chronic potassium depletion. As an alternative, deoxycorticosterone (DOC) may be used in a dose of 10 mg intramuscularly 12 hourly for 3 days. An oral load of 120 mmol of sodium chloride per 24 h for 4 days, added to the normal diet, will render hypokalaemic those 20% of patients with primary hyperaldosteronism who exhibit a normal serum potassium level. Differentiation of primary hyperaldosteronism caused by adenoma of the adrenal cortex from those cases due to hyperplasia depends, not only on the absolute level of plasma aldosterone (>830 pmol/L in adenoma), but also on the response of plasma aldosterone to postural changes (rising with the vertical posture in the case of hyperplasia, but not with adenoma).

FLUORESCEIN DILAURATE (PANCREOLAURYL, International Laboratories Ltd) TEST[5]

Principle

Pancreas-specific cholesterol ester hydrolase hydrolyses orally administered fluorescein dilaurate (bound fluorescein) in the small intestine, thus releasing free (unbound) fluorescein. The latter is then absorbed and excreted in the urine, where its measurement provides a quantitative assessment of pancreatic digestion. Bound fluorescein (i.e. unhydrolysed fluorescein) is not measured.

Indication

This is a useful screening test for identifying exocrine pancreatic insufficiency at an early stage.

Patient Preparation

The patient must avoid taking vitamins and pancreatic enzyme preparations for several days and should fast overnight. The test may be used for in-patients or out-patients. Smoking is not permitted.

Protocol

Following a breakfast of 20 g of butter with bread and (if desired) weak, unsweetened tea or coffee, without milk, a capsule of bound fluorescein is administered orally. The bladder is emptied and the urine discarded. All further urine is collected into a plain polythene bottle over the next 10 h and water intake (1 L over the next 2 h) encouraged. There should be no eating or drinking for the next 3 h after the capsule has been swallowed. On the following day, the whole procedure is repeated, but this time using a capsule of unbound fluorescein.

Sample Handling

Both of the 10 h samples of urine are estimated for unbound fluorescein.

Normal Response

An index is calculated using the excretion values obtained following ingestion of both the bound and free fluorescein preparations. The control collection following unbound fluorescein administration allows for individual variation in absorption and excretion. The excretion following the test capsule (containing the bound fluorescein) is expressed as a percentage of that following the control capsule (containing unbound fluorescein). In the normal subject >30% of the bound sample should be hydrolysed.

Interpretation

A value for the index of <20% is indicative of exocrine pancreatic insufficiency. Variable responses of 20–30% are sometimes found in chronic pancreatitis; such values would be an indication for repeating the test. False negative results are rare.

Comment

The fluorescein used in retinal angiography must be avoided prior to performing this test. The test is neither recommended in children, nor in women during pregnancy.

FORMIMINOGLUTAMIC ACID (FIGLU) TEST

Principle

Dietary L-histidine is converted to formiminoglutamic acid (FIGLU), which is then removed from the tissues by reacting with tetrahydrofolic acid. In the presence of folate deficiency, FIGLU cannot be metabolised; a large quantity, therefore, is excreted in the urine unaltered, measurement of which indicates the extent of folate depletion.

Indication

This test is indicated in patients with suspected folate deficiency, when measurements of serum and particularly red cell folate are not available.

Patient Preparation

The patient fasts overnight up to the start of the test. Smoking is not permitted.

Protocol

The early morning urine sample is discarded and a 24 h urine collection commenced into a polythene bottle containing 2 ml concentrated hydrochloric acid (care) and a few crystals of thymol. Breakfast is taken and 30 min later L-histidine (5 g) is administered orally, followed by further doses of 5 g each after both lunch and evening meal. It is necessary to mix well the insoluble L-histidine with orange juice and to drink it quickly, rinsing the cup 2 or 3 times, in order to ensure that the entire dose has been taken. A modified test in which the whole 15 g L-histidine is given in one dose is sometimes used, in which case the urine is collected for 8 h.

Sample Handling

This is as for FIGLU estimation in urine.

Normal Response

The 24 h FIGLU excretion should total $<200\ \mu$mol/24 h. In the modified test $<100\ \mu$mol/8 h is excreted.

59

Formiminoglutamic acid test

Interpretation

A FIGLU excretion of >200 μmol/24 h is observed in patients with folate deficiency, but also occurs in vitamin B_{12} deficiency, many forms of liver disease and malignancy in the absence of folate deficiency. In the modified test, a FIGLU excretion of >100 μmol/8 h is abnormal.

Comment

This test has been very largely replaced by direct estimation of folate in serum and especially in red cells, the latter being the best guide to body stores.

FRUCTOSE TOLERANCE TEST

Principle

Hereditary fructose intolerance (HFI) is characterised by fructose-1-phosphate aldolase deficiency, which results in intracellular accumulation of fructose-1-phosphate. The latter is thought to inhibit glycogenolysis and gluconeogenesis, and results in marked hypoglycaemia and hypophosphataemia following a fructose load, together with a high plasma fructose level and consequent fructosuria.

Indication

This test is indicated in both children and adults with suspected HFI. The beneficial response to restriction of sucrose, sorbitol and fructose (including fruit) intake from both diet and medications, should have been assessed previously.

Patient Preparation

The patient should not have eaten fruit or products containing fructose or its precursors for several weeks, must fast overnight and during the test, and should remain at rest in bed. Smoking is not permitted.

Protocol

Fructose (200 mg/kg body weight for both adults and children) is administered intravenously as a 20% w/v solution (i.e. a concentration of 20 g fructose/100 ml water), over 2–4 min. Venous blood (10 ml) is collected before the injection, and at 10 min intervals thereafter for 1 h, and then at 30 min intervals for a further 1 h, and apportioned between a glass bottle containing fluoride/oxalate, a plain polythene bottle and a bottle containing cold perchloric acid for plasma glucose, serum phosphate and blood lactate (special collection, see Appendix III) estimations respectively. Prior to the injection, the bladder is emptied and the urine discarded. All urine for the next 4 h is collected into a plain polythene bottle.

Sample Handling

This is as for estimation of plasma glucose, serum phosphate and

61

Fructose tolerance test

blood lactate, and qualitative detection in the urine of fructose.

Normal Response

The plasma glucose, serum phosphate and blood lactate should show little change and remain within the reference ranges. Fructose should not appear in the urine.

Interpretation

In HFI there is a fall in serum phosphate by approximately 0.5 mmol/L at 10 min, a fall in plasma glucose by approximately 2 mmol/L at 30 min, and a slow rise of blood lactate. Fructose may be detected qualitatively in the urine, but this may also occur as a lone feature in benign fructosuria, which may accompany advanced liver failure.

Comment

This is an important test for the confirmation of HFI. Unlike the oral fructose tolerance test, which it has replaced, the side effects are not unpleasant for either healthy subjects or patients with HFI; such effects are minimal, consisting merely of transient abdominal discomfort, the cause of which is obscure. In type I glycogen storage disease (von Gierke's disease), due to deficiency of glucose-6-phosphatase, the plasma glucose concentration determined every 10 min for 1 h fails to rise in this test; there is, however, a rapid rise in blood lactate. In other types of glycogen storage disease there is a normal rise in plasma glucose, but without elevation of blood lactate.

GALACTOSE TOLERANCE TEST

Principle

Galactose is metabolised in the liver to glucose. In the presence of liver failure this process is impaired, leading to high plasma levels of galactose following an intravenous load.

Indication

This test is indicated in patients with suspected liver failure, even in the absence of jaundice. It may be used sequentially in order to assess progress of the disease. **Caution: this test is contraindicated in galactosaemia.**

Patient Preparation

The patient fasts overnight and during the test. Smoking is not permitted.

Protocol

The bladder is emptied, following which galactose (500 mg/kg body weight), as a 50% w/v solution (i.e. a concentration of 50 g galactose/100 ml water) is administered intravenously over 4–5 min. Venous blood (5 ml) is collected into glass bottles containing fluoride/oxalate at 0, 45, 60, 75 and 120 min.

Sample Handling

This is as for estimation of plasma galactose.

Normal Response

The plasma galactose should be <5.4 mmol/L at 45 min, <2.3 mmol/L at 60 min and undetectable at 75 and 120 min.

Interpretation

Assuming normal renal function, elevated plasma galactose levels in this test are found in liver failure but also occur in hyperthyroidism.

Comment

This test replaces the oral galactose tolerance test which was less precise and more variable due to uncertainties of intestinal absorption; it was, therefore, less valuable for sequential quantification of liver function. In type I glycogen storage disease (von Gierke's disease), intravenous administration of galactose fails to cause the normal rise in plasma glucose.

63

GLUCAGON STIMULATION TEST
For glycogen storage diseases

Principle

Glucagon mobilises glucose from glycogen in the liver, but fails to do so normally in patients with certain types of glycogen storage disease.

Indication

This test is valuable in differentiating suspected glycogen storage diseases types I (von Gierke's disease), II (Pompe's disease) and III (Cori's limit dextrinosis).

Patient Preparation

The patient fasts overnight and remains at rest in bed. Smoking is not permitted, and there must be no eating during the test. In suspected type III glycogen storage disease, the test should be repeated in the recent post-prandial state, following 3 days on a high carbohydrate diet of 300 g daily.

Protocol

Glucagon (1 mg) is administered intramuscularly. Venous blood (5 ml) is collected at 0, 15 and 30 min into separate glass bottles, and apportioned between one containing fluoride/oxalate for plasma glucose estimation, and another containing cold perchloric acid for blood lactate estimation (special collection, see Appendix III).

Sample Handling

This is as for estimation of plasma glucose and blood lactate.

Normal Response

There should be a >50% rise in plasma glucose at 15–30 min following the glucagon injection, but no change in blood lactate.

Interpretation

In type I glycogen storage disease, which presents in infancy with fasting hypoglycaemia, there is no rise in plasma glucose in response to glucagon, either in the fasting or non-fasting state, but there is a further increase in the already elevated blood lactate. In type III glycogen storage disease, which also presents with fasting hypoglycaemia, there is similarly no rise in fasting plasma glucose following intramuscular glucagon, but there is a significant rise in the non-fasting state. In type II glycogen storage disease, in which fasting hypoglycaemia does not occur, there is a normal rise in plasma glucose after glucagon in both the fasting and non-fasting states; this is similar to the other glycogen storage diseases, except for types VI (Her's disease) and IV (Anderson's amylopectinosis), the latter showing a variable response depending on the degree of liver damage.

Comment

This test should normally be performed as one in a series of investigations, including the response to subcutaneous adrenaline, which should give similar results. Intravenous infusion of galactose or fructose differentiates type I glycogen storage disease from all the others.

GLUCAGON STIMULATION TEST
For growth hormone (GH) deficiency

Principle

Glucagon stimulates growth hormone (GH) release from the anterior pituitary gland. Following administration, glucagon causes elevation of serum GH levels, measurements of which serve as a test of anterior pituitary function.

Indication

This screening test is used in suspected GH deficiency, especially when the 'Insulin stress test' for hypothalamic-pituitary (anterior) assessment is considered dangerous, e.g. in children, or in adults with ischaemic heart disease or epilepsy.

Patient Preparation

The patient should be investigated under 'basal conditions' (see Appendix I), except that there is no restriction on water intake.

Protocol

Glucagon (1 mg for adults; 0.5 mg for children) is given either subcutaneously or intramuscularly, and venous blood (5 ml) is collected at 0, 60, 90, 120, 180, 210 and 240 min after the injection into plain glass bottles. Propranolol (40 mg) may be given orally to adults 2 h before the test in order to enhance the response to glucagon; however, this is not given to children. An intravenous catheter, inserted 30 min prior to collection of the first blood sample, should be used.

Sample Handling

This is as for serum GH estimation.

Response

There is a rise in serum GH from <10 mIU/L to >20 mIU/L, or a rise of >7 mIU/L at 2–3 h.

Interpretation

Failure to achieve the normal rise at any point indicates GH deficiency, either as part of panhypopituitarism, or because of selective deficiency. The chances of obtaining a false negative response are reduced when propranolol is used.

Comment

Local reaction, hypersensitivity, nausea and vomiting may complicate glucagon administration. In addition, the side effects and contraindications of propranolol should be noted. Glucagon is only one of several factors known to increase GH release; these include L-arginine, Bovril, clonidine, L-dopa and insulin.

GLUCAGON STIMULATION TEST
For insulinoma

Principle

Parenteral administration of glucagon promotes an increase in plasma glucose and a transient rise in serum insulin, not only secondary to the hyperglycaemia, but also because of a direct effect on the β-cells of the islets of Langerhans. The insulin release is exaggerated and prolonged in patients with insulinoma.

Indication

This test is useful for excluding insulinoma as the cause of demonstrated hypoglycaemia.

Patient preparation

The patient fasts overnight and throughout the test, remaining in bed. Smoking is not permitted. The patient should have received a high carbohydrate diet containing at least 300 g/day for 3 days prior to the test.

Protocol

Glucagon (30 μg/kg body weight, up to a maximum dose of 1 mg) is administered intramuscularly. Venous blood (5 ml) is collected and apportioned between glass bottles containing fluoride/oxalate and plain glass bottles at 0, 5, 10, 15, 20, 30, 60, 120 and 180 min following the glucagon injection.

Sample Handling

This is as for plasma glucose and serum insulin estimation.

Normal Response

The plasma glucose normally rises by >50% at 15–30 min, with subsequent return to basal (but not hypoglycaemic) levels. The serum insulin concentration rises in 5–20 min by approximately 30–100 mIU/L.

Interpretation

In some patients with insulinoma, a normal rise of plasma glucose

68

occurs, but there is a subsequent fall to hypoglycaemic levels. Serum insulin levels rise markedly above normal up to 500 mIU/L in 70% of cases of insulinoma, but marked rises may also be seen in patients with insulin resistance, e.g. obesity, acromegaly, and Cushing's syndrome. Glucose/insulin ratios are more informative than either value alone. A normal response is useful evidence against the presence of an insulinoma.

Comment

This test is more useful in excluding insulinoma than in making a positive diagnosis. Glucagon is structurally similar to secretin and is sometimes used in place of secretin in the 'Secretin stimulation test' for gastrinoma.

GLUCOSE-INSULIN PROVOCATION TEST

Principle

Administration of glucose together with insulin normally promotes the passage of extracellular potassium into cells. In patients with hypokalaemic periodic paralysis, this shift is exaggerated; there is, in consequence, a marked fall in serum potassium, accompanied by an episode of muscle weakness.

Indication

This test is useful for confirming the diagnosis of hypokalaemic periodic paralysis in patients in whom episodic muscle weakness is a feature. It is not necessary to perform this test in patients with demonstrated base-line hypokalaemia. Hyperthyroidism should have been excluded previously.

Patient Preparation

The patient should have received a high carbohydrate diet (300 g/ 24 h) for 3 days prior to the test, and is encouraged to take exercise. Potassium supplements should have ceased. **Caution: this may be hazardous.** Potassium-containing foods and drinks must be avoided; in addition, a high sodium chloride intake (150 mmol/24 h) is required for the 2 days prior to the test. These measures alone may precipitate an attack of muscle weakness, thereby confirming the diagnosis. Prior to the test the patient should fast overnight; this needs to continue throughout the procedure, with the patient remaining at rest in bed. Smoking is not permitted. Facilities for mechanical support of respiration should be at hand in the event of development of respiratory weakness; potassium chloride should be available for intravenous administration. **Caution: assuming renal function to be normal, the maximum concentration of potassium ion (K^+) for intravenous administration must not exceed 40 mmol/L, and the rate of infusion should not exceed 80 mmol/24 h given at a constant rate. Serum potassium should be monitored, bearing in mind that there is no overall depletion of body potassium.**

Protocol

Glucose (100 g) should be administered intravenously over 1 h as a

70

10% w/v solution (i.e. a concentration of 10 g glucose/100 ml water), containing 20 units of soluble insulin, i.e. a total volume of 1 L. Hypoglycaemic symptoms should not occur. The electrocardiogram (ECG) should be monitored at intervals for hypokalaemic changes. Venous blood (5 ml) should be collected into a plain glass bottle prior to commencing the infusion and also at 30, 60, 90, 120 and 240 min, and at any other time should muscle weakness develop.

Sample Handling

This is as for serum potassium estimation. Serum should be separated from red cells without delay.

Normal Response

There should be a fall in the serum potassium, but only within the reference range. Muscle weakness should not develop, and there should be no ECG changes.

Interpretation

A severe and either prolonged or transient fall in serum potassium from well within or at the lower limit of the reference range, with or without clinical features of muscle weakness (including respiratory involvement), favours the diagnosis of hypokalaemic periodic paralysis. Changes in the ECG may indicate myocardial involvement.

Comment

The patient should remain under observation for at least 24 h following the test. This procedure is not relevant in the diagnosis of either hyperkalaemic or normokalaemic periodic paralysis.

GLUCOSE TOLERANCE TEST (GTT)[6]
Intravenous procedure

Principle

Following a standard intravenous injection of glucose, it is found that plasma glucose levels over a defined period lie on an approximately straight line when plotted semi-logarithmically against time. From the slope obtained calculation of the glucose assimilation coefficient (K_g) can be made; this represents the assimilation of glucose by the tissues.

Indication

This test is essentially a research procedure. It is, however, of some value in establishing the diagnosis of diabetes mellitus in patients with intestinal malabsorption. Furthermore, it is occasionally used to make quantitative comparisons, not only in the same subject from time to time, but also between different subjects or groups of subjects.

Patient Preparation

The patient should be receiving a diet containing at least 150 g carbohydrate per day for 3 days prior to the test, and should fast overnight and remain at rest in bed. Smoking is not permitted.

Protocol

Glucose (50 ml) is administered as a sterile 50% w/v solution (i.e. a concentration of 50 g glucose/100 ml water) intravenously over a 2–4 min period. Venous blood (2.5 ml) is collected into glass bottles containing fluoride/oxalate at 10, 20, 30, 40, 50 and 60 min following the injection of glucose.

Sample Handling

This is as for plasma glucose estimation (performed by a glucose specific method).

Normal Response

The 20–60 min values are plotted on semi-logarithmic graph paper. Calculation of the K_g value from the glucose half-life in the blood in minutes ($t/2$) is made using the formula $K_g = 69.3/(t/2)$, which in the normal subject is 1.0–3.0.

Interpretation

In diabetes mellitus the K_g value is always <0.9 and usually <0.5. In athletes, higher values of the order of 5.0 may be obtained.

Comment

This test is of no value in the investigation of patients with hypoglycaemia. It is not a commonly used procedure.

GLUCOSE TOLERANCE TEST (GTT)
Oral procedure

Principle
Following a standard oral dose of glucose, plasma and urine glucose are monitored at regular intervals in the oral 'Glucose tolerance test (GTT)', in order to measure tolerance under defined conditions.

Indication
This test is indicated in patients with suspected impaired glucose tolerance (fasting plasma glucose 6.4–7.8 mmol/L), with particular reference to excluding diabetes mellitus (fasting plasma glucose >7.8 mmol/L) at an early stage. This suspicion may be aroused on the basis of clinical symptoms, demonstrated fasting hypergly-caemia or a 2 h post-prandial plasma glucose level of >11.1 mmol/L on a single occasion; the detection of glycosuria is not diagnostic of either impaired glucose tolerance or diabetes mellitus, as it can also occur in some normoglycaemic individuals. A prolonged oral 'GTT' for up to 5 h is helpful in the diagnosis of reactive hypoglycaemia.

Patient Preparation
The patient should not have been receiving drugs which affect glucose tolerance for the 2 weeks preceding this test. The oral 'GTT' should not be performed on seriously ill patients, including those with recent myocardial infarction and those showing metabolic response to trauma and surgery. The patient should receive a diet containing at least 150 g carbohydrate per day for 3 days prior to the test, and should not have been at rest in bed. The patient fasts overnight and during the test, but drinks at least 0.5 L of water during the previous evening, in order to ensure adequate urine production in the morning. The test can be performed as either an in-patient or out-patient procedure. Only light exercise is allowed, and smoking is not permitted.

Protocol
The bladder is emptied completely just prior to commencing the test and an aliquot of urine saved in a plain container. An oral glucose load of 75 g for adults (1.75 g/kg body weight for children, up to a maximum of 75 g) is given under supervision, well dissolved in a

glass of water flavoured with lemon juice and drunk over 2–3 min, care being taken to avoid vomiting at any stage. Venous blood (2.5 ml) is collected into glass bottles containing fluoride/oxalate at 0, 30, 60, 90 and 120 min. Further aliquots of urine are collected at each complete emptying of the bladder at 60 and 120 min. If a prolonged oral 'GTT' is being performed, further blood samples should be taken similarly at 3, 4 and 5 h, with additional venous blood (2.5 ml) being placed into plain glass bottles at these times for serum insulin estimation.

Sample Handling

This is as for estimation of plasma glucose (performed by a glucose specific method), urine glucose (performed without delay) and ketones, and serum insulin levels where required.

Normal Response

There should be a base-line plasma glucose concentration of <6.4 mmol/L with a rise to <10.0 mmol/L at 30 min, and a return to <7.8 mmol/L by 120 min. No glucose should appear in the urine. Serum insulin levels in the prolonged oral 'GTT' should be appropriate to the plasma glucose concentrations.

Interpretation

Glycosuria in the presence of a normal plasma glucose level indicates either a low renal threshold for glucose or a renal tubular defect. Glycosuria, in the presence of normoglycaemia, is frequently encountered in pregnancy. A marked and prolonged rise in plasma glucose of greater than the reference values is a feature of diabetes mellitus. The many other causes of impaired glucose tolerance including pancreatic disease should be excluded, especially if ketonuria and acidosis are absent. A flat plasma glucose curve is a feature of generalised intestinal malabsorption, hypopituitarism, adrenocortical insufficiency and primary hypothyroidism, but may also be seen in young athletes; non-compliance by the patient, vomiting shortly after the glucose load and delay in gastric emptying can sometimes be the explanation of a 'flat curve'. A 'lag curve' is seen after gastrointestinal surgery, in thyrotoxicosis and in severe liver disease, but this, too, may occur in normal individuals. In essential reactive hypoglycaemia, a prolonged oral 'GTT' (up to 5 h) gives limited support to this diagnosis by the demonstration of low plasma glucose levels later than 2 h after the load (with inappropriately high serum insulin levels), insulinoma having been previously excluded. Drugs which decrease glucose tolerance include corticosteroids, oral contraceptives, thiazides and sympathomimetic agents. Other drugs may have a similar effect in overdosage.

Comment

The oral 'GTT' is of no value in assessing the progress of diabetes mellitus, and the demonstration of clearly raised glucose levels at any time, if repeated, renders the test superfluous. The cortisone-stressed 'GTT' is now obsolete. The 'Growth hormone (GH) suppression test', based on the oral 'GTT', is used in the diagnosis of active acromegaly or gigantism, in which there is a paradoxical response characterised by a rise of serum GH.

GONADOTROPHIN-RELEASING HORMONE (Gn-RH, luteinizing hormone/follicle-stimulating hormone-releasing hormone, LH/FSH-RH) STIMULATION TEST

Principle

Gonadotrophin-releasing hormone (Gn-RH, luteinizing hormone/follicle-stimulating hormone-releasing hormone, LH/FSH-RH) is a hypothalamic decapeptide; administration of the synthetic preparation results in synthesis of both luteinizing hormone (LH) and follicle-stimulating hormone (FSH) within the anterior pituitary gland and their secretion into the blood. This release is abnormal, not only in disorders of the hypothalamus and anterior pituitary gland, but also in primary disorders of the gonads.

Indication

This test is of value in suspected hypothalamic/pituitary disease, constitutional delayed puberty in males, and in primary gonadal failure. It may comprise part of the investigation regimens for infertility and amenorrhoea.

Patient Preparation

No special preparation is essential, but ideally the patient should fast overnight and during the test, and be at rest in bed. Smoking is not permitted. Repeat tests (if required) should be carried out at the same time of day.

Protocol

Gn-RH (100 μg) is given intravenously. Venous blood (5 ml) is collected into plain glass bottles at 0, 20 and 60 min following the injection.

Sample Handling

This is as for serum LH and FSH estimation.

Normal Response

In adults, serum LH shows at least a 2- to 4-fold increase, with maximum value being at 20 min. Serum FSH shows a 2- to 3-fold increase, also with maximum value at 20 min. In children, the FSH response may exceed the LH response.

Interpretation

An exaggerated response from a high resting level is seen in patients with primary testicular disease, e.g. Kleinfelter's syndrome. An impaired response suggests anterior pituitary disease or constitutional delayed puberty. In the early stages of the polycystic ovary syndrome (PCOS), the basal serum LH is only slightly elevated, but there is an exaggerated response in this test; later, there is more marked elevation of serum LH compared with the FSH and the serum testosterone is also raised. A normal response does not necessarily exclude hypothalamic/ pituitary disease. Differentiation between hypothalamic and pituitary disease may only become apparent after repeated testing, failure of response suggesting the latter. Patients with severe generalised illness may also show an impaired response.

Comment

This test is used frequently either as part of a combined test of pituitary reserve function, or by itself. The other test often required in conjunction with this is the 'Human chorionic gonadotrophin (HCG) stimulation test'.

GROWTH HORMONE (GH) SUPPRESSION TEST

Principle

In the presence of either active acromegaly or gigantism, the normal suppression of growth hormone (GH) by food or glucose does not occur. The patient, therefore, exhibits a high basal serum GH level, which may rise even further in response to a standard oral glucose load.

Indication

The test is of value in confirming the presence of active acromegaly or gigantism, particularly in the early stages.

Patient Preparation

This is as for the oral 'Glucose tolerance test (GTT)'. The patient should not be receiving GH-stimulating drugs.

Protocol

This is as for the oral 'GTT'.

Sample Handling

This is as for estimation of both plasma and urine glucose; serum samples are collected as for GH.

Normal Response

The normal response is for serum GH to be suppressed to <3 mIU/L at some point during the period of the test.

Interpretation

In patients with active disease, there is failure of a high resting serum GH to suppress and indeed there may be a paradoxical rise. Often there is also evidence of decreased glucose tolerance. A paradoxical rise may also occur in renal failure and diabetes mellitus. Failure of suppression is sometimes seen in advanced liver disease, heroin addiction and anorexia nervosa.

Comment

This is a useful test for confirming suspected early acromegaly, or for establishing whether or not obvious acromegaly is still active. In 'burnt out' acromegaly, the basal serum GH level returns gradually towards normal, although impaired glucose tolerance may persist.

HEPARIN TEST

Principle

Lipoprotein lipase of tissue origin is released into the blood following a small bolus injection of heparin intravenously. Low activity of plasma lipoprotein lipase following heparin administration is a feature of several conditions, but particularly Fredrickson type I hyperlipoproteinaemia (familial hyperchylomicronaemia, the chylomicronaemia syndrome) by definition.

Indication

This test may be used for confirming the diagnosis of Fredrickson type I hyperlipoproteinaemia.

Patient Preparation

The patient should receive a normal diet for 3–4 days and should then fast overnight prior to the test. Smoking is not permitted.

Protocol

Heparin (10 units/kg body weight) is injected intravenously. Venous blood (5 ml) is collected for estimation of plasma lipoprotein lipase (special collection, see Appendix III) into glass bottles containing sodium citrate prior to and 10 min following the injection.

Sample Handling

This is for estimation of plasma lipoprotein lipase activity.

Normal Response

The 10 min post-heparin plasma lipoprotein lipase activity is 240–520 U/L.

Interpretation

Very low plasma lipoprotein lipase activity following heparin injection is diagnostic of Fredrickson type I hyperlipoproteinaemia, though the range of activity in this condition lies between 60 and 710 U/L. Levels in the upper part of this range do not, therefore, exclude the diagnosis. Low plasma lipoprotein lipase activity is also seen in hypothyroidism, diabetes mellitus, liver disease, severe alcoholism, renal failure, pancreatitis and Fredrickson type V hyperlipoproteinaemia (exogenous hypertriglyceridaemia, mixed hyperlipoproteinaemia).

Comment

This is a specialised test and is not routinely required for the diagnosis of Fredrickson type I hyperlipoproteinaemia. Some authors have advocated the use of inhibitor substances to differentiate hepatic from non-hepatic sources of lipoprotein lipase.

HUMAN CHORIONIC GONADOTROPHIN (HCG) STIMULATION TEST

Principle

Administration of human chorionic gonadotrophin (HCG) causes a rise of serum testosterone in prepubertal boys and adult males, and a rise of serum 17α-hydroxyprogesterone and oestradiol in the latter as well. Measurement of these hormones reflects testicular Leydig cell reserve and functional capacity.

Indication

The short version of this test (see below) is useful for differentiating constitutionally delayed puberty from hypogonadism secondary to hypothalamic-pituitary disease. The prolonged version of the test (see below) is indicated in the diagnosis of primary gonadal failure in children, in whom serum follicle-stimulating hormone (FSH) and luteinizing hormone (LH) levels have not yet risen, e.g. cryptorchidism (unilateral or bilateral), anorchia and in some cases of pseudo-hermaphroditism. It is also occasionally indicated in females with suspected polycystic ovary syndrome (PCOS). This test is not indicated in hypogonadism associated with elevated basal levels of serum FSH or LH.

Patient Preparation

No special preparation is required for the test, which may be performed on in-patients or out-patients.

Protocol

In the short version, HCG (2000 IU) is administered intramuscularly as a single injection, and venous blood (10 ml) is collected into plain glass bottles at time 0, at 2–4 h, and daily thereafter for 5 days. In the prolonged version, HCG (2000 IU) is injected intramuscularly at least twice at intervals of 3–4 days with venous blood (10 ml) being collected into plain glass bottles prior to and at 48 h following each injection.

Sample Handling

This is as for serum testosterone, 17α-hydroxyprogesterone and oestradiol estimation.

Normal Response

In the short version, there should be an initial 1.5-fold increase in the serum testosterone in adult males at 2–4 h reflecting liberation of stored steroid, followed by a fall. A later rise between the second and fourth day of up to 2- to 4-fold reflects Leydig cell biosynthetic function. In the prolonged version, adult males show a modest rise of serum testosterone together with elevation of serum 17α-hydroxyprogesterone and oestradiol. Prepubertal boys show no response of 17α-hydroxyprogesterone and oestradiol, but exhibit a marked rise of serum testosterone.

Interpretation

Patients with constitutionally delayed puberty show a marked rise in serum testosterone in response to HCG administration, particularly in the prolonged version, whilst those with gonadotrophin deficiency as a consequence of hypothalamic-pituitary disease, show an impaired response. Patients with primary gonadal deficiency, e.g. pseudohermaphroditism and anorchia, fail to respond. Ovarian steroid production following HCG administration in normal females is low, but is somewhat increased in the PCOS.

Comment

This test, when required, should be carried out after a 'Gonadotrophin-releasing hormone (Gn-RH, luteinizing hormone/ follicle-stimulating hormone-releasing hormone, LH/FSH-RH) stimulation test'. Impaired release of testosterone in both tests points to gonadotrophin deficiency of organic origin. In renal failure, there is decreased testosterone response to HCG.

HYDROCORTISONE SUPPRESSION TEST

Principle

Hydrocortisone suppresses hypercalcaemia, probably by antagonising the action of vitamin D.

Indication

This test may be indicated in order to elucidate the cause of hypercalcaemia (especially if marked) in patients with suspected primary or tertiary hyperparathyroidism. It is particularly useful in excluding hyperparathyroidism from the other causes of hypercalcaemia, notably sarcoidosis in which there is marked vitamin D sensitivity.

Patient Preparation

No special preparation is required. This test can be performed on either in-patients or out-patients.

Protocol

Hydrocortisone (40 mg) is administered orally 8 hourly every day for 10 days, and withdrawn gradually over the next 5 days. Venous blood (5 ml) is collected without stasis into plain glass bottles from the fasting patient on the 2 days immediately prior to commencing the test, and also on days 5, 8 and 10. **Caution: the patient should be observed for the effects of fluid retention and the test avoided in those with heart failure.**

Sample Handling

This is as for serum calcium and albumin estimation.

Normal Response

This test is not performed in healthy subjects in whom there is a normal serum calcium level. It is used for differentiating the causes of hypercalcaemia.

Interpretation

Of all patients with primary (and tertiary) hyperparathyroidism, 90% show no significant suppression of serum calcium during this test, and it is in these patients in whom the test is most useful. A marked reduction of serum calcium by 0.5–1.0 mmol/L is seen in 60% of patients showing hypercalcaemia associated with sarcoidosis, and also in ectopic parathyroid hormone (PTH) production by malignant tumours. Exceptions to this suppression are advanced malignant disease of bone, and severe hyperthyroidism, neither of which, however, is a clinically difficult diagnostic problem. Patients with hyperparathyroidism who do show suppression of serum calcium usually have significant bone involvement. A marked fall in serum calcium in this test occurs in vitamin D intoxication.

Comment

The test is particularly valuable when hypercalcaemia is marked. In the interpretation of results, allowance must be made for fluid retention during the period of steroid administration by relating total serum calcium to the albumin concentration. This test is only rarely indicated, as in most cases of marked hypercalcaemia the diagnosis is made on the basis of other criteria; in those in whom the hypercalcaemia is slight, the test is of least value. An alternative procedure is to administer prednisone or prednisolone (10 mg) orally 8 hourly for the 10 days of the test.

85

HYDROGEN BREATH TEST[7]

Principle

Disaccharidase deficiencies lead to the presence of excessive amounts of residual carbohydrate in the lower intestinal tract. Bacterial action on this residual carbohydrate leads to the production of increased quantities of free hydrogen, which diffuses through the body tissues and is excreted in the breath. This process is exacerbated in the presence of an oral load of a specific disaccharide. Bacterial overgrowth in the small intestine is also associated with increased breath hydrogen following oral glucose administration.

Indication

This test is indicated in any patient suspected of having a primary disaccharidase deficiency, particularly that of lactase; in adults it is used mainly for the purpose of identifying small intestinal bacterial overgrowth.

Patient Preparation

The patient fasts overnight and throughout the test and should be seated in a chair for the procedure. Smoking is not permitted.

Protocol

A specific disaccharide, e.g. lactose, maltose, sucrose (1 g/kg body weight), is administered in water orally when the test is used for identifying disaccharidase deficiencies; glucose (1 g/kg body weight), a monosaccharide, is administered in the same manner when the test is used in patients suspected of having small intestinal bacterial overgrowth. End-tidal expired air (the last 25% of exhaled breath) is collected using a 20 ml syringe with a three-way tap. Samples are collected prior to administration of the carbohydrate and at 15 min intervals thereafter for a period of 2 h.

Sample Handling

Expired air is estimated for hydrogen content.

Normal Response

In the normal subject there is a low breath hydrogen content of <10 parts per million (ppm) and a negligible increase following the carbohydrate load.

Interpretation

In the disaccharidase deficiencies there is a progressive rise in breath hydrogen throughout the 2 h period to levels >20 ppm and usually considerably more. Increased content is also noted in patients with marked gastrointestinal hurry, and false positive results may occur with bacterial overgrowth in the small intestine, e.g. blind loop syndrome. Negative results occur, even in patients with disaccharidase deficiencies, if hydrogen-producing bacteria are not present in the intestine, particularly following oral antibiotic therapy. Following administration of a glucose load, an early rise in breath hydrogen lends support to the diagnosis of small intestinal bacterial overgrowth.

Comment

This test is rapidly becoming a standard procedure. It has the advantage over the ^{14}C-lactose breath test of not involving use of radioactive isotopes; it also measures the total small bowel digestive and absorptive capacity. Inability to perform forced expiration, as in elderly subjects, does not invalidate the test.

HYPOTHALAMIC-PITUITARY (ANTERIOR) FUNCTION (COMBINED HYPOTHALAMIC-RELEASING HORMONE/INSULIN) TEST

Principle

This test constitutes a stress reaction to rapidly produced hypo-glycaemia of significant degree which, together with stimulation by injected hypothalamic-releasing hormones, permits, via blood hormone measurements, assessment of hypothalamic-anterior pituitary reserve function. Estimation in the blood of the pituitary hormones, namely adrenocorticotrophic hormone (ACTH), growth hormone (GH), thyroid-stimulating hormone (TSH), luteinizing hormone (LH), follicle-stimulating hormone (FSH) and prolactin (PRL), together with cortisol and glucose, forms the basis of the test.

Indication

This test is useful in assessing suspected hypothalamic-pituitary insufficiency. **Caution: this test is dangerous, especially in children and is contraindicated in patients with epilepsy, ischaemic heart disease and primary adrenocortical insufficiency.**

Patient Preparation

Any replacement thyroxine therapy should be discontinued 5 days prior to the test and replacement steroids 12 h before the test. **Caution: this may be hazardous.** Dopamine-blocking drugs which raise serum PRL levels should not have been taken for at least 2 weeks prior to the test. The patient should be investigated under 'basal conditions' (see Appendix I), except that there is no restriction on water intake. At least 30 min should be allowed to elapse following insertion of an intravenous catheter before collecting the baseline blood samples. The test should be performed in the morning.

Protocol

Soluble insulin (0.15 units/kg body weight) is the standard dose given intravenously; a smaller dose (0.05 units/kg body weight) is used when hypopituitarism is suspected and a larger dose (0.30 units/kg body weight) when insulin resistance is anticipated, e.g. in acromegaly, Cushing's disease and obesity. The soluble insulin is followed immediately by 200 μg thyrotrophin-releasing hormone (TRH) and 100μg gonadotrophin releasing-hormone (Gn-RH, luteinizing hormone/follicle-stimulating hormone-releasing hormone, LH/FSH-RH), also given intravenously and mixed as a bolus injection in 5 ml sterile water. If symptomatic hypoglycaemia has not occurred 45 min (see below) after the injection of insulin, a further dose of 50% of the amount given should be administered at this stage, sample timings recommencing at this point, for plasma ACTH, and serum cortisol and GH. Venous blood (20 ml) is collected at 0, 20, 30, 45, 60, 90 and 120 min and divided between polythene bottles containing heparin, plain glass bottles, and glass bottles containing fluoride/oxalate for estimation of plasma ACTH (special collection, see Appendix III), serum cortisol, GH, TSH, LH, FSH and PRL and plasma glucose respectively. Following the test, the patient is given a carbohydrate-rich meal and observed carefully, especially for the next 2 h. Though not generally recommended, this test may be performed on out-patients, in which case 5 mg prednisone should be given orally at the end of the procedure. If steroid treatment has been withdrawn, 100 mg hydrocortisone should be given intravenously prior to recommencing steroid therapy. Caution: great vigilance is necessary throughout the test for evidence of severe and prolonged hypoglycaemia, which may occur as early as 15–30 min. Should symptoms of prolonged hypoglycaemia occur, these are likely to be due to hypoglycaemic unresponsiveness; glucose (20 ml), as a sterile 50% w/v solution (i.e. a concentration of 50 g glucose/100 ml water) may then be required to be given intravenously, but this will not invalidate the test. Rarely, pituitary apoplexy is a subsequent complication.

Sample Handling

This is as for estimation of plasma ACTH, serum cortisol, GH, TSH, LH, FSH and PRL and plasma glucose.

Normal Response

It is necessary for the plasma glucose to fall to <2.2 mmol/L for this test to be valid; it should return to the reference range by 30 min. There should be a marked rise in the measured pituitary and target organ hormones, with the different responses peaking at 20–90 min.

The degree of the various responses varies widely, and reference range limits (particularly for the peak responses) should not be regarded too rigidly (see Table, Appendix IV).

Interpretation

Adequate hypoglycaemia (plasma glucose <2.2 mmol/L) must be induced. An impaired response may be either overall or selective, e.g. selective GH deficiency in some types of dwarfism, and selective LH/FSH deficiency in Kallman's syndrome. High basal levels of serum cortisol, PRL and GH may indicate a stress reaction, and high PRL levels alone may be due to a prolactinoma or pituitary stalk lesion which leads to loss of prolactin-inhibitory factor (PIF). Some pituitary tumours may produce several hormones in excess. In panhypopituitarism all anterior pituitary hormones and serum cortisol fail to rise normally. Failure of serum GH to rise may be seen in primary hypothyroidism. All the responses must be considered together and viewed carefully in light of the whole clinical context of the patient before final conclusions are drawn as to the assessment of hypothalamic-anterior pituitary reserve function.

Comment

The test is uncomfortable for the patient. Measurements of plasma ACTH may well be omitted if there are difficulties in performing the assay; serum cortisol will suffice on the assumption that adreno-cortical function is intact. Insulin is only one of several factors known to increase GH release; these include L-arginine, Bovril, clonidine, L-dopa and glucagon. Other tests of anterior pituitary function include the 'Insulin stress test' for hypothalamic-pituitary (anterior) assessment and the 'Pituitary (anterior) function (combined hypothalamic-releasing hormone/ arginine vasopressin) test'.

INSULIN STRESS TEST
For hypothalamic-pituitary (anterior) assessment

Principle

The stress of insulin-induced hypoglycaemia, rapidly produced and of sufficient degree, stimulates, via the hypothalamus, release of growth hormone (GH), adrenocorticotrophic hormone (ACTH) and prolactin (PRL) from the anterior pituitary gland. Measurement of these hormones in the blood, together with estimation of appropriate target organ hormones, permits assessment of hypothalamic-anterior pituitary reserve function.

Indication

This test is used as the standard provocative stimulus for assessing reserve function of GH and ACTH, and can also be used for PRL studies. **Caution: this test is dangerous, especially in children, and in contraindicated in patients with epilepsy, ischaemic heart disease and primary adrenocortical insufficiency.**

Patient Preparation

Any replacement steroid therapy should be discontinued 12 h prior to the test. **Caution: this may be hazardous.** Dopamine-blocking drugs which raise serum PRL levels should not have been taken for at least 2 weeks prior to the test. The patient should be investigated under 'basal conditions' (see Appendix I), except that there is no restriction on water intake. At least 30 min should be allowed to elapse following insertion of an intravenous catheter before collecting the base-line blood samples. The test should be performed in the morning.

Protocol

Soluble insulin (0.15 units/kg body weight) is the standard dose given intravenously; 0.05 units/kg body weight is appropriate if marked hypopituitarism is suspected, and 0.3 units/kg body weight if insulin resistance is anticipated, e.g. in acromegaly, Cushing's disease and obesity. If symptomatic hypoglycaemia has not occurred 45 min (see below) after the injection of insulin, a further dose of 50% of the amount given should be administered at this stage, sample timings recommencing at this point. Venous blood

91

(20 ml) is collected at 0, 20, 30, 45, 60, 90 and 120 min and divided between polythene bottles containing heparin, plain glass bottles, and glass bottles containing fluoride/oxalate for estimation of plasma ACTH (special collection, see Appendix III), serum cortisol, GH and PRL and plasma glucose respectively. Following the test, the patient should be given a carbohydrate-rich meal and observed carefully, especially for the next 2 h. Though not generally recommended, this test may be performed on out-patients, in which case 5 mg prednisone should be given orally at the end of the procedure. If steroid treatment has been withdrawn, 100 mg hydrocortisone should be given intravenously prior to recommencing steroid therapy. **Caution: great vigilance is necessary throughout the test for evidence of severe and prolonged hypoglycaemia, which may occur as early as 15–30 min. Should symptoms of prolonged hypoglycaemia occur, these are likely to be due to hypoglycaemic unresponsiveness; glucose (20 ml), as a sterile 50% w/v solution (i.e. a concentration of 50 g glucose/100 ml water) may then be required to be given intravenously, but this will not invalidate the test. Rarely, pituitary apoplexy is a subsequent complication.**

Sample Handling
This is as for estimation of plasma ACTH, serum cortisol, GH and PRL and plasma glucose.

Normal Response
It is necessary for the plasma glucose to fall to <2.2 mmol/L for this test to be valid. It should return to the reference range by 30 min. There should be a marked rise in the measured pituitary and target organ hormones (see Table, Appendix IV) with the different responses peaking at 20–90 min. The degree of the various responses varies widely, and reference range limits (particularly for the peak responses) should not be regarded too rigidly.

Interpretation
Adequate hypoglycaemia (i.e. plasma glucose <2.2 mmol/L) must be induced; impaired hormonal response to this may be overall or selective. High basal levels of serum GH, cortisol and PRL may indicate a stress reaction. High serum PRL levels alone may be due to a prolactinoma or a pituitary stalk lesion. Levels of plasma ACTH,

and serum cortisol, GH and PRL will fail to rise normally in hypopituitarism. Failure of serum GH levels to rise may be due to primary hypothyroidism. All the responses must be considered together and viewed carefully in light of the whole clinical context of the patient before final conclusions are drawn as to the assessment of hypothalamic-anterior pituitary reserve function.

Comment

This test is uncomfortable for the patient. Measurements of plasma ACTH may well be omitted if there are difficulties in performing the assay; serum cortisol will suffice on the assumption that adrenocortical function is intact. Insulin is only one of several factors known to increase GH release; these include L-arginine, Bovril, clonidine, L-dopa and glucagon. Other tests of anterior pituitary function include the 'Hypothalamic-pituitary (anterior) function (combined hypothalamic-releasing hormone/insulin) test' and the 'Pituitary (anterior) function (combined hypothalamic-releasing hormone/arginine vasopressin) test'.

INSULIN STRESS (HOLLANDER) TEST
For vagotomy assessment

Principle
This test is based on the knowledge that hypoglycaemia induces gastric acid secretion via the vagus nerve.

Indication
This test is used post-operatively to assess the completeness of vagotomy in patients with persisting gastrointestinal symptoms.

Patient Preparation
The patient fasts overnight and on the day of the test and remains at rest in bed. Smoking is not permitted.

Protocol
A nasogastric tube is passed as in the 'Pentagastrin stimulation test' for gastric acid secretion. Overnight (residual) juice is aspirated and discarded, and basal (resting) juice is then collected for 60 min. Soluble insulin (0.2 units/kg body weight) is given subcutaneously and venous blood (2.5 ml) collected at 0, 15, 30, 45 and 60 min. Gastric aspirate is collected at 15 min intervals into separate plain glass bottles for a further 1 h after the insulin injection. Close supervision of the patient is necessary, with sterile 50% glucose w/v (i.e. a concentration of 50 g glucose/100 ml water) being available for intravenous injection in case of severe hypoglycaemia. This test is best performed 3–6 months after vagotomy; it should not be performed in the first 2 weeks after surgery.

Sample Handling
This is as for estimation of gastric acid secretion and plasma glucose.

Normal Response
Vagotomy is regarded as complete if there is no significant gastric acid secretion in the presence of a plasma glucose level of <2.5 mmol/L accompanied by symptoms of hypoglycaemia.

94

Interpretation

Failure to produce gastric acid in the presence of demonstrated hypoglycaemia indicates, but does not absolutely confirm, completeness of vagotomy. However, the presence of small amounts of gastric acidity does not exclude total vagotomy, on account of the occurrence of non-vagal hormonal stimulation of gastric acid.

Comment

This test is uncomfortable for the patient, and it is rarely necessary to perform it more than once.

INULIN CLEARANCE TEST

Principle

Inulin is an inert material, being neither absorbed nor excreted by the renal tubules. It is cleared quantitatively by the renal glomerulus, thus providing a reliable measure of the glomerular filtration rate (GFR).

Indication

This is essentially a research procedure for quantitation of glomerular filtration in adequately hydrated, non-oedematous patients.

Patient Preparation

The patient should be well hydrated with 1 L of water administered orally 1 h before the test, having fasted overnight and remaining at rest in bed. Smoking is not permitted.

Protocol

Inulin (25 ml of a sterile 10% solution, i.e. 10 g inulin/100 ml water) is injected intravenously, followed by an infusion of 500 ml of a 1.5% solution of inulin (i.e. 1.5 g inulin/100 ml water) given at a rate of 4 ml/min in order to maintain a constant blood concentration. The bladder is emptied 30 min after the initial dose and the urine discarded. Three urine collections are made thereafter at 20 min intervals during the next hour, each being placed into a plain glass bottle. Venous blood (5 ml) is collected into a plain glass bottle at the beginning and end of the 1 h urine collection period. Measurement is made of the patient's height and weight in order to permit calculation of body surface area.

Sample Handling

This is as for estimation of serum and urine inulin.

Normal Response

The inulin clearance is 125±40 ml/min/1.73 m^2. It is reduced in children and elderly subjects.

Interpretation

The clearance is increased in hypermetabolic states and in pregnancy. It is decreased in low output cardiac failure, shock and renal impairment.

Comment

This is an accurate test but is not suitable for routine use. It serves as a reference for other clearance tests. Determination of inulin is a difficult procedure.

IRON ABSORPTION TEST

Principle

In the presence of iron deficiency, a significant rise in serum iron, following oral administration of a standard dose of a readily absorbable inorganic iron salt, excludes malabsorption of iron as the cause.

Indication

This is a useful test in patients with low serum iron and hypochromic anaemia, in order to determine whether or not the condition is correctable by administering oral iron supplements.

Patient Preparation

The patient fasts overnight and during the test.

Protocol

Venous blood (5 ml) is taken into a plain glass bottle prior to and 2 h after an oral dose of powdered ferrous sulphate (100 mg) has been given in water.

Sample Handling

This is as for serum iron estimation.

Normal Response

A 2- to 3-fold increase in serum iron occurs, particularly if the initial value is low. Estimation of urinary iron excretion following oral administration is not diagnostically useful.

Interpretation

Failure of serum iron to rise indicates defective iron absorption.

Comment

Foods and liquids with a high tannin or phytate content inhibit the absorption of iron; vitamin C aids absorption. A low serum iron level does not necessarily indicate failure of absorption or body depletion of iron. Serum ferritin is a better index of the body iron stores than is serum iron. Hypochromic anaemia is usually, but not necessarily, associated with iron deficiency; the thalassaemias and sideroblastic anaemias are characterised by normal or elevated serum iron.

ISCHAEMIC EXERCISE TEST

Principle
Severe exercise of the forearm muscles, of short duration and under conditions of ischaemia, fails to promote the normal rise in blood lactate in patients with several types of generalised muscle glycogen storage disorder, particularly type V glycogen storage disease (McArdle's disease), due to myophosphorylase deficiency. This is on account of specific muscle enzyme deficiencies in the anaerobic phase of glycolysis in these disorders.

Indication
The test is used in patients with suspected muscle glycogen storage disease, especially in young adults with progressive muscular pain and cramps on exercise.

Patient Preparation
The patient is admitted preferably overnight, and must be investigated under 'basal conditions' (see Appendix I). The patient should be totally inactive but should empty the bladder for comfort 1 h before commencement of blood sampling.

Protocol
A base-line venous blood sample (5 ml) is collected from the antecubital vein of one arm via a needle or intravenous catheter, without stasis, for blood lactate estimation (special collection, see Appendix III). A sphygmomanometer cuff is placed around the wrist (cuff 1) and another high on the upper arm of the same side (cuff 2). Cuff 1 is inflated to about 200 mmHg, to prevent collateral circulation to the arm muscles via the deep arterial anastomosis in the hand. Cuff 2 is inflated to above the systolic blood pressure and the forearm muscles exercised vigorously by opening and closing the fist forcefully for 45 seconds, timed with a stop-watch or until prevented by pain or muscle contracture. Cuff 2 is then deflated and further blood samples are taken at 1, 2, 5 and 7 min after finishing the exercise, cuff 1 remaining inflated throughout. Further blood samples may then be taken at 10 and 15 min with both cuffs deflated. Accurate timing, particularly of the early blood samples, is essential, the exact moment of venepuncture being recorded by means of a stop-watch.

99

Sample Handling

The bottles are sent to the laboratory for re-weighing at room temperature, followed by estimation of blood lactate in the supernatant after centrifugation.

Normal Response

The basal venous blood lactate should be <1.8 mmol/L, followed by a marked rise to >2.5 mmol/L in the first 5 min with a sharp peak at between 1 and 3 min.

Interpretation

Failure of the blood lactate to rise is characteristic of McArdle's disease, but is also a feature of phosphoglucomutase, phosphohexoseisomerase, phosphofructokinase and acid maltase deficiency; it is also seen in some lipid storage disorders of muscle. Apparent failure of blood lactate to rise may occur if the 1 min sample is inaccurately timed or if the patient fails to exercise adequately.

Comment

This is a very useful test for excluding the above rare disorders; all these conditions may exhibit myoglobinuria following vigorous generalised exercise. Measurement of plasma ammonia (special collection, see Appendix III), in response to ischaemic forearm exercise, has been advocated as an additional parameter, exaggerated levels having been described in McArdle's disease.

LACTOSE TOLERANCE TEST

Principle

Lactase deficiency in the small intestine leads to lactose intolerance and consequent failure of the blood glucose to rise normally following ingestion of lactose-containing products, particularly milk.

Indication

This test is useful in patients with suspected primary lactase deficiency. It should not be carried out in patients with diabetes mellitus on account of difficulty in interpretation. **Caution: the test may cause abdominal discomfort and diarrhoea.**

Patient Preparation

The patient fasts overnight and during the test and should remain at rest in bed. Smoking is not permitted.

Protocol

Lactose (1 g/kg body weight) is administered orally in 400 ml of water. Venous blood (5 ml) is collected at 0, 15, 30, 60, 90 and 120 min into plain glass bottles containing fluoride/oxalate.

Sample Handling

This is as for plasma glucose estimation.

Normal Response

The plasma glucose should rise by at least 1.1 mmol/L, but usually by >1.67 mmol/L.

Interpretation

Lactase deficiency, whether primary (congenital) or secondary (to gastrointestinal resection or disease, e.g. malabsorption syndromes), is confirmed by a plasma glucose rise of <1.1 mmol/L and the spontaneous complaint of symptoms relating to abdominal discomfort, borborygmi, flatulence and diarrhoea. Failure of plasma glucose to rise adequately may also be due to non-compliance by the patient, vomiting of the test dose or delayed gastric emptying.

101

Comment

Lactase deficiency is common in non-Caucasians. Temporary lactase deficiency may be encountered in the premature infant. Other disaccharidase deficiencies include sucrose and maltose intolerance, and these may be diagnosed by observing response to the appropriate carbohydrate load. The detection of more than one type of carbohydrate intolerance suggests, but does not prove, the presence of generalised mucosal disease. Confirmation of lactase or other disaccharidase deficiencies depends on per-oral jejunal biopsy, followed by measurements of the activities of various disaccharidases. Detection of lactose in the urine is helpful in confirming the diagnosis of lactase deficiency; the 'Hydrogen breath test' is also useful.

L-LEUCINE SENSITIVITY TEST

Principle

Oral administration of L-leucine causes excessive insulin release in children with leucine sensitivity and in subjects of any age who are taking sulphonylurea drugs or who suffer from insulinoma.

Indication

This test is useful in cases of suspected hypoglycaemia, especially in children, some of whom may present with severe hypoglycaemia following the ingestion of casein (which contains L-leucine).

Patient Preparation

The patient should receive a diet containing at least 4 g/kg body weight of carbohydrate daily for 3 days prior to the test, must fast both overnight and during the test, and should remain at rest in bed.

Protocol

L-Leucine (150 mg/kg body weight for adults and children) is administered orally in water. Venous blood (2.5 ml) is collected at 0, 15, 30, 45, 90, 120, 150 and 180 min into plain glass bottles and bottles containing fluoride/oxalate.

Sample Handling

This is as for plasma glucose and serum insulin estimation.

Normal Response

There should be a fall in plasma glucose by < 1.5 mmol/L or by < 50% of the fasting level at any stage, together with a rise of serum insulin of < 30 mU/L.

Interpretation

Demonstration of hypoglycaemia in response to L-leucine is suggestive of leucine sensitivity, but it may also be seen in patients receiving sulphonylurea drugs and in those with insulinoma, especially if high serum insulin levels are also present. In the absence of demonstrated hypoglycaemia, insulin values are difficult to interpret. A normal response, however, does not exclude the presence of an insulinoma, but this test is not primarily used for establishment of this diagnosis. A negative response is expected in reactive hypoglycaemia.

Comment

This test is currently less frequently used than formerly. Leucine sensitivity tends to be a self-limiting condition.

LUNDH TEST[8]

Principle

A standard test meal of carbohydrate, protein and fat stimulates liberation of secretin and cholecystokinin-pancreozymin (CCK-PZ) from the duodenal mucosa. This, in turn, results in stimulation of exocrine pancreatic secretion, which may be assessed by measurement of tryptic activity in the aspirated duodenal contents.

Indication

This test is used for the assessment of exocrine pancreatic function in patients with suspected chronic pancreatitis or carcinoma of the head of the pancreas.

Patient Preparation

The patient fasts overnight and during the test and remains at rest in bed. Smoking is not permitted.

Protocol

A radio-opaque double lumen tube of internal diameter >2 mm is passed, the tip being placed in the fourth part of the duodenum under radiological control. Confirmation of the correct location is obtained by an initial aspiration demonstrating the pH of the fluid to be alkaline. A meal, consisting of 18 g corn or soya bean oil, 15 g Casilan and 40 g glucose, homogenised in hot water and made up to 300 ml, is administered in the form of a drink, following which the patient reclines. The external end of the tube is placed in a measuring cylinder (chilled in ice) below the level of the duodenum. Fluid is collected by siphonage for the next 2 h as four 30 min samples, which are sent to the laboratory immediately to be frozen at – 20 °C; aspiration may be required. Complete collection of all the duodenal contents is not necessary.

Sample Handling

The specimens should be pooled in the laboratory and mixed well prior to estimation of tryptic activity. It is permissible to store the aspirate at – 20 °C for up to 4 weeks.

Normal Response

The normal mean tryptic activity of duodenal aspirate is 17 IU/L, with a minimum of 6 IU/L.

Interpretation

This test is positive for pancreatic insufficiency, as assessed by a tryptic activity of <6 IU/L, in 67% of cases of chronic pancreatitis and in some 80% of cases of carcinoma of the head of the pancreas. Weak false positive responses are seen in 25% of patients with coeliac disease due to diminished enzyme release from the atrophic mucosa and also in long-standing diabetes mellitus, duodenal ulcer and following partial gastrectomy.

Comment

The test is simpler to perform and more physiologically relevant than the 'Secretin/cholecystokinin-pancreozymin (CCK-PZ) stimulation test'. It should not be performed following gastric surgery.

L-METHIONINE LOAD TEST

Principle

In patients with homocystinuria, in whom there is cystathionine synthetase deficiency, L-methionine (either in the diet or following administration for diagnostic purposes) is poorly metabolised. This results in high and prolonged plasma levels of L-methionine, with consequent increased excretion of homocystine in the urine.

Indication

The test may be used in patients with suspected homocystinuria when the classical diagnostic biochemical feature (i.e. positive nitroprusside test in the urine) is absent or equivocal, especially in mild cases of late onset in adolescence or even the early twenties.

Patient Preparation

The patient fasts overnight prior to and for the duration of the test but is encouraged to drink water throughout.

Protocol

L-Methionine (100 mg/kg body weight) is given orally in a flavoured drink over a period of 5 min (methionine is rather insoluble and possesses an unpleasant taste); 250 mg tablets of L-methionine are also available. Immediately prior to the dose, the bladder is emptied and the urine discarded, but for the next 6 h all urine is collected into a plain glass bottle. In addition, venous blood (2 ml) is collected into a glass bottle containing heparin at time 0 and hourly for 6 h for plasma L-methionine and homocystine estimation.

Sample Handling

This is as for estimation of plasma and urine amino acids and for the nitroprusside test in urine. The plasma sample must be dispatched to the laboratory immediately. For the nitroprusside test a fresh urine sample is required.

Normal Response

There is normally a rapid fall in plasma L-methionine following attainment of the peak level. No homocystine is found in plasma or urine. There is a negative nitroprusside test in the urine.

Interpretation

In homocystinuria, there is a marked rise and slow fall in the concentration of L-methionine in plasma; in addition, homocystine is present in excess in both plasma and urine. A negative nitroprusside test does not exclude the diagnosis; a positive test, however, is found in both homocystinuria and cystinuria. This test gives variable results in heterozygotes. Some other very rare conditions may give rise to homocystine in the urine.

Comment

L-Methionine does not appear in more than negligible amounts in the urine on account of reabsorption in the renal tubules.

METYRAPONE (METOPIRONE) STIMULATION TEST

Principle

Metyrapone blocks 11β-hydroxylase activity in the adrenal cortex, this being the last step in cortisol synthesis. The consequent decrease in cortisol normally stimulates the feedback mechanism to the hypothalamus and anterior pituitary gland, resulting in increased production of ACTH. This, in turn, stimulates production of steroids up to 11-deoxycortisol (compound S), which may be measured directly in the serum or indirectly in the urine as 17-oxogenic steroids (17-OGS). In hypothalamic/pituitary disease there is failure of this response.

Indication

This test may be used to assess decreased anterior pituitary reserve function associated with organic disease or following prolonged therapy with adrenocortical steroids. It can also be of assistance in the differential diagnosis of Cushing's syndrome.

Patient Preparation

The patient should be in hospital for this test and at rest in bed, with provision being made for dealing with induced acute adrenocortical insufficiency, especially in children. Glucocorticoid preparations or oestrogen therapy should not have been administered for several days prior to this test.

Protocol

Two 24 h urine collections in plain polythene bottles are commenced 2 days prior to administration of the first dose of metyrapone. Metyrapone (500–750 mg) is administered orally to adults 4-hourly for 6 doses according to weight. Three further 24 h urine collections are commenced immediately after the first dose of the compound. Venous blood (25 ml) is collected into a plain glass bottle for serum 11-deoxycortisol and cortisol determination and a polythene bottle containing heparin for plasma ACTH determination (special collection, see Appendix III), at time 0 and on day 4, both samples being collected at the same time of day. Caution: this test may be dangerous in children due to precipitation of acute adrenocortical insuf-

109

ficiency; it may also be dangerous in subjects who are to undergo anaesthesia or surgical procedures shortly afterwards. The test is contraindicated in pregnancy and primary renal failure.

Sample Handling
This is as for estimation of serum 11-deoxycortisol, cortisol (by a specific method), plasma ACTH and urine 17-OGS.

Normal Response
There should be a rise in serum 11-deoxycortisol and a moderate fall in serum cortisol, together with a marked rise in plasma ACTH during the test. There should be a 2–6 fold increase over the base-line urinary excretion of 17-OGS.

Interpretation
In primary adrenocortical insufficiency (Addison's disease), which is associated with a high plasma ACTH and low serum cortisol, there is no response in this test, i.e. there is no rise in serum 11-deoxycortisol, or urinary 17-OGS excretion following metyrapone administration. In the absence of primary adrenocortical failure, an impaired response indicates secondary adrenocortical failure (hypothalamic/pituitary insufficiency), due either to organic disease or to prolonged corticosteroid therapy; the consequent low plasma ACTH is due either to inability of hormone elaboration, or to impaired hypothalamic-pituitary activation via negative feedback control. In pituitary-dependent Cushing's disease associated with high plasma ACTH, adrenocortical hyperplasia and high serum cortisol, there is an exaggerated response of the urine 17-OGS to metyrapone. In Cushing's syndrome, due to either an adrenal adenoma or an ectopic ACTH-producing tumour (associated with low and high plasma ACTH respectively), there is an impaired response of the urine 17-OGS to metyrapone, despite the high initial serum cortisol levels in both.

Comment
Drugs which interfere with this test include enzyme-inducing agents (e.g. anticonvulsants, oestrogens and glucocorticoids), opium alkaloids and phenothiazines. The test is useful, but time-consuming and is less used nowadays. A shorter modified out-patient test has been described but is less satisfactory.

OLEIC ACID AND TRIOLEIN ABSORPTION TEST

Principle

Intestinal absorption of triolein is dependent upon pancreatic lipase, whilst oleic acid absorption is independent of this enzyme. Both fail to be absorbed in non-pancreatic malabsorption.

Indication

The test is used to confirm the diagnosis of intestinal malabsorption and to differentiate pancreatic from non-pancreatic causes.

Patient Preparation

On the evening before the test, 10 drops of Lugol's iodine solution are given in order to saturate the thyroid gland, thus preventing uptake of isotope. The patient fasts overnight. Smoking is not permitted.

Protocol

^{131}I-Triolein (1850 kBq, 50 μCi) and ^{125}I-oleic acid (1850 kBq, 50 μCi) are given orally with milk. Venous blood (10 ml) is collected into heparin tubes at 4 and 6 h. All stools are collected for 72 h.

Sample Handling

Blood and all stools are sent to the laboratory for differential counting of ^{131}I and ^{125}I in both the plasma and total stool sample.

Normal Response

Approximately 1.7% or more of the total radioactive dose administered should be found per litre of plasma at 4 and 6 h. Less than 5% of the total radioactivity administered should be found in the stool over the 72 h collection.

Interpretation

The finding of decreased levels of both isotopes in the blood suggests malabsorption of non-pancreatic origin, including that due to increased intestinal mobility. Normal, or near normal, absorption of ^{125}I-oleic acid in the presence of decreased absorption of ^{131}I-triolein suggests pancreatic malabsorption. In pancreatic

111

disease, 20–30% of the ^{131}I-triolein administered may be found in the stool, but there is only slightly increased ^{125}I-oleic acid content.

Comment

The ^{131}I-triolein administered in this test is hydrolysed during the normal digestive process. Hydrolysis of unabsorbed ^{131}I-triolein by colonic bacteria limits the usefulness of stool estimations; nevertheless, a combination of plasma and stool counts is better than either alone. An alternative test is the ^{14}C-triolein absorption test in which the absorbed labelled glycerol is metabolised by the liver to $^{14}CO_2$, which is exhaled and measured in the breath.

D-PENICILLAMINE CHELATION TEST

Principle

D-Penicillamine (D-β, β-dimethylcysteine), following oral administration, chelates the excess copper, which is loosely bound to tissue
protein in patients with Wilson's disease (hepato-lenticular de-
generation). There is thus enhanced excretion of copper in the
urine.

Indication

This test is an aid to the diagnosis of Wilson's disease, of either
predominantly hepatic or neurological type.

Patient Preparation

No special preparation is required, apart from avoiding foods with
high copper content (e.g. chocolate, liver, mushrooms, shell-fish
and nuts) for a few days prior to and during the test.

Protocol

Two 24 h urine collections are made commencing 2 days prior to
administration of the D-penicillamine; these serve as a base-line.
Adult patients are given D-penicillamine (500 mg) orally, 8-hourly
for 3 days, in the form of tablets. In the case of children, assuming
average height and weight, the total daily dose (divided 8-hourly)
for 16, 12, 6, 4 and 2 years of age is respectively 1 g, 800 mg, 500 mg,
400 mg and 300 mg. Three further 24 h urine samples are collected
during D-penicillamine administration. All urine is collected and
stored in specially prepared copper-free, acid-washed, polythene
bottles for estimation of copper excretion (special collection, see
Appendix III).

Sample Handling

This is as for 24 h urine copper estimation. Particular care must be
taken to avoid contamination of the samples with traces of copper.

Normal Response

The base-line 24 h urine copper excretion in adults should be < 1.25
μmol/24 h. Following D-penicillamine administration, no specimen

113

should possess a copper content in excess of 18 μmol/ 24 h.

Interpretation

A base-line urine copper excretion >1.25 μmol/24 h and >18 μmol/ 24 h in any other sample is suggestive but not diagnostic of Wilson's disease.

Comment

The results by no means establish firmly the diagnosis of Wilson's disease but are useful when taken in conjunction with other evidence. The upper limit of the reference range is more precisely defined for the base-line excretion than for that following D-penicillamine administration. All these urine studies are, therefore, of great importance in the urgent diagnosis of this serious progressive disorder, which is amenable to treatment. Occasionally, there may be an anaphylactic reaction to D-penicillamine and/or a sudden marked reduction in the platelet count: however, the latter is rare during the short-term administration required for diagnostic purposes, as compared with the long-term administration needed in the treatment of Wilson's disease. Estimation of both basal serum copper and urinary copper excretion are the appropriate tests used for assessing not only compliance, but also response to treatment.

PENTAGASTRIN STIMULATION TEST
For calcitonin (CT) release

Principle

Pentagastrin stimulates excessive release of calcitonin (CT) into the circulation of patients with medullary carcinoma of the thyroid gland (MCT).

Indication

The test is of value in patients with suspected MCT in the absence of diagnostically high plasma CT levels. It is particularly helpful in the screening of family members of a known case.

Patient Preparation

The patient fasts overnight and remains at rest in bed. Smoking is not permitted.

Protocol

Pentagastrin (0.5 μg/kg body weight), available as a solution of 500 μg/2 ml, is administered intravenously. Venous blood (10 ml) is collected into polythene bottles containing heparin pre-cooled on ice at 0, 1, 2, 5 and 10 min following the injection, for plasma CT estimation (special collection, see Appendix III).

Sample Handling

This is as for plasma CT estimation; samples should be processed immediately. Visible haemolysis invalidates the results.

Normal Response

Normal base-line levels of plasma CT are <100 ng/L in males and <50 ng/L in females. In males there is a rise in plasma CT to <200 ng/L following the pentagastrin injection, whereas in females there is a smaller rise to <100 ng/L.

Interpretation

Following the pentagastrin injection, an excessive rise in plasma CT, starting from normal levels, is suggestive of occult MCT.

Comment

Pentagastrin is only one of several factors known to increase CT release; others include calcium and whisky.

115

PENTAGASTRIN STIMULATION TEST[9]
For gastric acid secretion

Principle
Pentagastrin is a synthetic analogue comprising the first 5 amino acids of gastrin. Both compounds stimulate gastric acid production.

Indication
This test is indicated in patients with persistent duodenal ulcer, some with pernicious anaemia and in any person suspected of having the Zollinger-Ellison syndrome. It may also be helpful in the diagnosis of carcinoma of the stomach and chronic gastritis. It is of little diagnostic value in the investigation of gastric ulcer.

Patient Preparation
The patient fasts overnight and during the test and remains at rest in bed. Smoking is not permitted.

Protocol
The patient is placed in a semi-recumbent position. A nasogastric tube is passed, preferably under radiological control, so that the tip lies in the gastric antrum. Continuous aspiration of the stomach contents is made for 1 h in order to obtain the basal (resting) juice, the overnight (residual) juice having already been discarded. An injection of pentagastrin (6 μg/kg body weight), available as a solution of 500 μg/2 ml, is given intramuscularly and aspiration made of all gastric juice at 15 min intervals during the post-stimulation period for a total of 1 h; specimens are collected separately into plain glass bottles. A basal venous blood sample (5 ml) is collected into a polythene bottle containing heparin and Trasylol, pre-cooled on ice, for plasma gastrin estimation (special collection, see Appendix III).

Sample Handling
The timed portions of gastric contents are sent to the laboratory without delay. Measurements of the volume, pH and total acidity of the gastric aspirates are made. The blood sample must be sent to the laboratory immediately.

116

Normal Response

The pre-stimulation sample and the 4 post-stimulation samples of gastric aspirate are measured separately for volume, pH and acid content. Acidity is expressed for the pre-stimulation specimen as mmol/h and for the post-stimulation specimens as mmol/15 min, in the first instance. The 2 highest values for acid content in the post-stimulation samples are then added together, multiplied by 2 and expressed as mmol/h, thus constituting the peak acid output (PAO). Alternatively, summation of the acid contents for each of the 4 post-stimulation samples, expressed as mmol/15 min, constitutes the maximal acid output (MAO). Normal values for volume and acid content of gastric juice are expressed below:

	Pre-stimulation (basal output)	Post-stimulation (maximal output)
Volume	10–90 ml/h	20–300 ml/h
pH	1.5–4.0	<1.5
Total acid secretion	0–5 mmol/h	20–40 mmol/h

The PAO, calculated as above, is normally 5–40 mmol/h.

Interpretation

Wide variations occur. Patients with duodenal ulcer characteristically have a high basal acidity (5–15 mmol/h) which rises, following stimulation with pentagastrin, to the order of 40 mmol/h, although figures >40 mmol/h suggest the possibility of the Zollinger-Ellison syndrome. In the latter there is a high basal gastric juice volume of >100 ml/h, together with high basal acidity and secretion (20–60 mmol/h) and high PAO (60–100 mmol/h), often with little difference between the basal and PAO values; in addition, the plasma gastrin level is high. The PAO is generally regarded as being a more valuable parameter than the MAO and is of use in determining the form of gastric surgery for duodenal ulcer. In gastric ulcer this test is of relatively little value. Achlorhydria, being characterised by a pH >6.0 is an essential feature of adult pernicious anaemia, but not of the juvenile form. Achlorhydria following insulin-induced hypoglycaemia is a feature of successful vagotomy.

Comment

This test is safer and has fewer side effects than the now-discarded augmented histamine test meal. It is important to examine the specimen of gastric aspirate for excessive blood and mucus, particularly in cases of achlorhydria with suspected malignancy. Pentagastrin is one of several factors known to increase CT release: others include calcium and whisky.

PENTOLINIUM TARTRATE SUPPRESSION TEST[10]

Principle

Failure of suppression of elevated plasma adrenaline and noradrenaline levels, following intravenous administration of the ganglion-blocking drug pentolinium tartrate, indicates autonomous production of catecholamines by a tumour, situated either within the adrenal medulla or elsewhere.

Indication

This test is indicated mainly for confirming the diagnosis of phaeochromocytoma in the presence of temporary or persistent elevation of plasma catecholamines.

Patient Preparation

The patent should not have received antihypertensive drugs for 7 days prior to this investigation. The test may be performed on either in-patients or out-patients. Smoking is not permitted. The subject should lie quietly in the supine position both prior to and following insertion of an intravenous catheter and should remain so for a further 1 h following administration of the hypotensive drug pentolinium tartrate. Checks of the blood pressure, in both supine and erect posture, are made at regular intervals. **Caution: the test involves all the possible hazards of induced hypotension including urinary suppression**

Protocol

Venous blood (5 ml) is collected into chilled glass bottles containing heparin, prior to, and at 10 and 20 min following intravenous administration of pentolinium tartrate (2.5 mg) as a bolus injection, for plasma adrenaline and noradrenaline estimation (special collection, see Appendix III).

Sample Handling

Blood samples are sent to the laboratory immediately and are centrifuged without delay at +4 °C. Plasma is stored at − 20 °C and estimated within 1 week for adrenaline and noradrenaline.

119

Normal Response

Plasma concentrations of catecholamines in all samples should lie within the reference ranges.

Interpretation

High base-line levels of plasma catecholamines may be due to anxiety, which can resemble phaeochromocytoma clinically; however, in this situation, the plasma catecholamines suppress in response to pentolinium tartrate. Failure of suppression of elevated base-line plasma catecholamines is strongly suggestive of an autonomous catecholamine-secreting tumour. The commonest type is a phaeochromocytoma, which may be located in the adrenal medulla or elsewhere. Such tumours may be single or multiple.

Comment

This is a specialised test requiring very accurate analysis of plasma catecholamines.

PHOSPHATE EXCRETION INDICES TEST

Principle

Renal phosphate excretion can be expressed as phosphate clearance (PC), phosphate/creatinine clearance ratio (Cp/Ccr), tubular reabsorption of phosphate (TRP) and phosphate excretion index (PEI). The latter three indices relate to creatinine clearance, thus minimising inaccuracies of urine collection, estimations of serum and urine phosphate, the effect of fluctuations in glomerular filtration rate with time, and the consequences of early impairment of glomerular function on the interpretation of renal tubular phosphate excretion.

Indication

This test is indicated in cases of suspected primary, secondary or tertiary hyperparathyroidism, hypoparathyroidism and renal tubular hyperphosphaturia.

Patient Preparation

A normal diet with respect to calcium and phosphate should be taken for 5 days prior to commencing the test. The patient fasts overnight and during the test, but is encouraged to drink water freely in the early morning on the day of the test (in order to ensure an adequate and constant urine output), and should remain at rest in bed except at the times of passing urine. Smoking is not permitted.

Protocol

The patient passes urine at (say) 9.00 am, emptying the bladder completely. This specimen is discarded. All urine is then collected for approximately 1 h (but precisely timed), at the end of which the bladder is again completely emptied; this time the specimen is collected into a plain glass bottle. The urine volume is noted and, if less than 60 ml, more water is drunk. Venous blood (10 ml) is collected into a plain glass bottle at approximately the half-way point, i.e. at 9.30 am. The process is completed for a second hour, with the accurately timed urine sample ending at approximately 11.00 am, with a further blood sample being collected at 10.30 am.

121

Sample Handling

This is as for both serum and urine phosphate and creatinine estimation. All samples must be sent to the laboratory as soon as complete; the urine volumes are measured. Serum should be separated from the blood cells soon after collection. Both serum and urine phosphate should be estimated on the same day as the samples are collected.

Normal Response

The PC is 6–15 ml/min, the Cp/Ccr ratio is 0.03–0.13, the TRP is 84–97% and the PEI is 0 ± 0.09.

Interpretation

The PC, Cp/Ccr ratio and PEI tend to be raised and the TRP reduced in primary, secondary or tertiary hyperparathyroidism and in renal tubular hyperphosphaturia. The PC, Cp/Ccr ratio and PEI tend to be reduced and the TRP raised in both hypoparathyroidism and pseudohypoparathyroidism.

Comment

These indices are less frequently required now that serum parathyroid hormone (PTH) assays are more freely available.

PITUITARY (ANTERIOR) FUNCTION (COMBINED HYPOTHALAMIC-RELEASING HORMONE/ARGININE VASOPRESSIN) TEST[11]

Principle

Hypothalamic-releasing hormones stimulate release of the corresponding pituitary hormones. Simultaneous administration of arginine vasopressin enhances the response of both cortisol and growth hormone (GH), when compared with that induced following administration of either the hypothalamic-releasing hormones or insulin alone. Measurements in the blood of the pituitary hormones, namely adrenocorticotrophic hormone (ACTH), growth hormone (GH), thyroid-stimulating hormone (TSH), luteinizing hormone (LH), follicle-stimulating hormone (FSH) and prolactin (PRL), together with cortisol, permit assessment of anterior pituitary reserve function.

Indication

This test is indicated in suspected anterior pituitary insufficiency, especially in patients in whom the 'Insulin stress test' for hypothalamic-pituitary (anterior) assessment is regarded as unsafe.

Patient Preparation

Any replacement thyroxine therapy should be discontinued 5 days prior to the test and replacement steroids 12 h before the test. **Caution: this may be hazardous.**Dopamine-blocking drugs, which raise serum PRL levels, should not have been taken for at least 2 weeks prior to the test. This test may be performed on either in-patients or out-patients, though the latter is not generally recommended. At least 30 min should be allowed to elapse after inserting an intravenous catheter before collecting the base-line blood sample. The test should be performed in the morning.

Protocol

Rapid sequential intravenous injections (over a period of 2 min) of 100 μg human corticotrophin-releasing factor (CRF), 100 μg GH-releasing hormone (GH-RH), 100 μg gonadotrophin-releasing hormone (Gn-RH, luteinizing hormone/follicle-stimulating hormone-releasing hormone, LH/FSH-RH), and 200 μg thyrotrophin-releasing hormone (TRH) are given. Arginine vasopressin (10 pressor units) is injected intramuscularly at the same time. Venous blood (10 ml) is collected at 0, 30, 60 and 90 min and is divided between polythene bottles containing heparin and plain glass bottles, for estimation of plasma ACTH (special collection, see Appendix III), and serum cortisol, GH, TSH, LH, FSH and PRL respectively.

Sample Handling

This is as for estimation of plasma ACTH, and serum cortisol, GH, TSH, LH, FSH, and PRL.

Normal Response

There should be a marked rise in the measured pituitary and target organ hormones (see Table, Appendix IV), with the different responses peaking at 20–90 min. The degree of the various responses varies widely, and reference range limits (particularly for the peak responses) should not be regarded too rigidly. The cortisol and GH responses are enhanced by the arginine vasopressin, and may be slightly greater than the figures quoted in the table.

Interpretation

An impaired response may be either over-all or selective. In partial panhypopituitarism the GH, LH and FSH responses are impaired early, whereas the TSH, ACTH and cortisol responses are affected later. High basal levels of plasma ACTH, serum cortisol, GH and PRL, if present, may represent a reaction to stress, though a high PRL level alone may be due either to a PRL-secreting tumour, i.e. prolactinoma (which may be a microtumour), or pituitary stalk lesion (which leads to loss of prolactin-inhibitory factor). Some pituitary tumours may produce several hormones in excess. Failure of serum GH to rise may be seen in primary hypothyroidism. This test assesses anterior pituitary function on a wide basis, and a rise of pituitary hormones in the blood of patients with the clinical features of hypothalamic/pituitary insufficiency points to a lesion of the pituitary stalk or hypothalamus, whereas failure of a rise points to a disorder of the pituitary gland, or of both the pituitary gland and hypothalamus; however, it should be borne in mind that many pituitary tumours have suprasellar extensions. Failure of the pituitary hormones to rise in either situation indicates the necessity for replacement therapy, but a rise in patients with a hypothalamic disorder alone does not indicate that replacement therapy is not necessary. All the responses must be considered together and viewed carefully in light of the whole clinical context of the patient before final conclusions are drawn as to the assessment of anterior pituitary reserve function.

Comment

The test is not uncomfortable for the patient and is generally regarded as safe, requiring less medical supervision than the 'Insulin stress test' for hypothalamic-pituitary (anterior) assessment, but the occurrence of pituitary apoplexy has been described as a rare complication following the procedure. Measurements of plasma ACTH may well be omitted if there are difficulties in performing the assay; serum cortisol will suffice on the assumption that adrenocortical function is intact. Other tests of anterior pituitary function include the 'Hypothalamic-pituitary (anterior) function (combined hypothalamic-releasing hormone/insulin) test' and the 'Insulin stress test' for hypothalamic-pituitary (anterior) assessment.

POTASSIUM LOAD TEST

Principle

Patients with hyperkalaemic periodic paralysis (adynamia episodica hereditaria) and normokalaemic periodic paralysis are not improved by oral potassium supplements, and indeed both are clinically intolerant of a potassium load, the former developing, in addition, a raised serum potassium. In these respects both disorders differ from hypokalaemic periodic paralysis and may be differentiated from this condition by administering a high intake of potassium salts.

Indication

This test is useful for diagnosis, both in patients with hyperkalaemic periodic paralysis, and in those who fall within the heterogeneous group of normokalaemic periodic paralysis. **Caution: it is vital to ensure that renal function is normal before administering oral potassium salts, which in any case might prove hazardous.**

Patient Preparation

The patient should receive a low sodium diet (<10 mmol/24 h) for 3 days prior to the test.

Protocol

Potassium (40 mmol) is given **orally** in divided doses in the form of a soluble salt with meals over the course of the day. If necessary, further doses are given on successive days, up to a maximum of 120 mmol potassium for the 3 days of the test. Venous blood (5 ml) is collected into a plain glass bottle prior to administration of the first dose of potassium, and thereafter daily for a further 3 days.

Sample Handling

This is as for serum electrolytes, serum being estimated for potassium.

Normal Response

The serum potassium concentration should remain within the reference range, and the subject should neither develop new symp-

126

toms, nor show clinical deterioration.

Interpretation

Patients with hyperkalaemic periodic paralysis demonstrate a rise in serum potassium above the upper limit of the reference range in association with symptoms of muscle weakness, stiffness and sometimes myotonia. Patients with normokalaemic periodic paralysis may demonstrate some or all of these features, but without elevation of serum potassium above the upper limit of the reference range.

Comment

This is a rarely used specialised test.

PROTEIN CLEARANCE (SELECTIVITY INDEX) TEST

Principle

In renal glomerular disease, associated with significant proteinuria of >2 g/day, comparison of the clearance of small molecular weight proteins such as transferrin (Tf) of molecular weight 81 000 daltons, with the clearance of larger molecular weight proteins such as immunoglobulin G (IgG) of molecular weight 155 000 daltons is helpful with respect to assessing the prognosis following corticosteroid therapy. Minimal change glomerulonephritis (one of the causes of the nephrotic syndrome), as opposed to advanced membranous glomerulonephritis, is characterised by 'leakage' of Tf rather than IgG into the urine, and carries a good prognosis, especially in children.

Indication

This test is indicated in early renal glomerular disease, particularly in children.

Patient Preparation

No special preparation is required.

Protocol

A random venous blood sample (5 ml) is collected into a plain glass bottle. A urine sample is collected at the same time, into a plain polythene bottle.

Sample Handling

Serum and urine are estimated for Tf and IgG, and the ratio of the clearances of both is calculated (IgG/Tf clearance ratio).

Normal Response

This test has no application to healthy subjects, in whom proteinuria is absent.

128

Interpretation

An IgG/Tf clearance ratio of < 0.2 in the presence of total proteinuria of >2 g/day is indicative of minimal change glomerulonephritis; a good prognosis with corticosteroid therapy is to be expected. A higher ratio suggests membranous glomerulonephritis, with poorer prognosis.

Comment

The IgG/Tf clearance ratio is independent of inaccuracies in urine collection. The test is of value in adults as well as in children, but the best predictive results are obtained in the latter group. An alternative procedure is to calculate the IgG/albumin clearance ratio.

SECRETIN STIMULATION TEST

Principle

Secretin stimulates the G-cells of a pancreatic gastrinoma, thus releasing gastrin. It does not, however, stimulate the G-cells located in the antrum of the stomach of either a normal subject or one with antral G-cell hyperplasia.

Indication

This test is useful in patients with suspected gastrinoma (Zollinger-Ellison syndrome), and for differentiating this from antral G-cell hyperplasia.

Patient Preparation

The patient fasts overnight and remains at rest in bed. Smoking is not permitted.

Protocol

Secretin (75 units) is administered slowly intravenously to adults over 2 min as a freshly prepared solution (available from AB Kabi Diagnostica, Nykoping, Sweden). Venous blood (10 ml) is collected into glass bottles containing heparin and Trasylol at − 5, 0, 5, 10, 20, 30, 45 and 60 min after the injection for plasma gastrin estimation (special collection, see Appendix III).

Sample Handling

This is as for plasma gastrin estimation; samples should be processed immediately.

Normal Response

There should be either a fall or no change in the plasma gastrin from the normal base-line level of <100 pmol/L.

Interpretation

A 2- to 3-fold rise in plasma gastrin suggests the presence of a gastrinoma, whereas a fall from a moderately raised base-line level suggests antral G-cell hyperplasia. Very high base-line plasma gastrin levels may be found in patients with hypochlorhydria from many causes; such levels suggest gastrinoma only if associated with high gastric acid output. A few false negative responses may occur.

Comment

A modification of this test is by giving the secretagogues as an intravenous infusion. Great attention must be paid to specificity and purity of the secretin preparation. Glucagon is structurally similar to secretin and sometimes replaces secretin in this test. An alternative stimulation procedure for gastrin release involves calcium infusion.

SECRETIN/CHOLECYSTOKININ-PANCREOZYMIN (CCK-PZ) STIMULATION TEST[9]

Principle

Secretin is a polypeptide occurring naturally in the mucosa of the upper small intestine. A preparation of this, when given intravenously in association with cholecystokinin-pancreozymin (CCK-PZ), also an upper intestinal polypeptide, stimulates the exocrine pancreas to secrete maximally. This response is assessed by analysing the duodenal aspirate for enzyme and bicarbonate content, and also by measuring its volume.

Indication

This test is used in cases of suspected exocrine pancreatic insufficiency, particularly when due to chronic pancreatitis. Though useful, also, in cases of pancreatic carcinoma, the test may give negative results with tumours in the tail of the pancreas. It is contraindicated in tumours of the head of the pancreas suspected of involving the common bile duct.

Patient Preparation

The patient fasts overnight and throughout the test, remaining at rest in bed. Smoking is not permitted.

Protocol

A double-lumen tube is passed under radiological control, one opening of which is positioned to enable continuous aspiration of the gastric contents, thus preventing admixture with the duodenal secretions. The latter are collected separately from the other lumen of the tube which is placed in the second part of the duodenum, close to the opening of the pancreatic duct. The overnight (residual) juice is discarded, but the basal (resting) juice is collected for two 10 min periods. Secretin (1–2 units/kg body weight) is given slowly intravenously over 2 min as a freshly prepared solution and 6 more 10 min samples are collected (secretin is available from AB Kabi Diagnostica, Nykoping, Sweden). CCK-PZ (1–2 units/kg body weight) is then given slowly intravenously over 5 min, also as a freshly prepared solution, followed by collection of 2 further 10 min samples (CCK-PZ is available from Ferring Pharmaceuticals Ltd).

Sample Handling

The duodenal aspirates are placed separately in ice-cooled plain glass bottles and sent immediately to the laboratory. The volumes are measured, and estimation made of tryspin, lipase, amylase and bicarbonate.

Normal Response

At maximal secretion, following the secretin stimulation, the volume of duodenal aspirate should be >2 ml/kg body weight/h, the bicarbonate concentration rising to >75 mmol/L. Following the CCK-PZ stimulation, there is a marked increase in enzyme activities of the duodenal aspirate.

Interpretation

This test is useful for confirming the presence of pancreatic disease, though it is less reliable in establishing the aetiology. Nevertheless, in chronic pancreatitis, at maximal secretion, the bicarbonate concentration of the duodenal aspirate is <80 mmol/L at an early stage in the disease, but with preservation of enzyme activities until later; these, however, eventually fall below the reference ranges. The volume is reduced to <2 ml/kg body weight/h. In carcinoma of the pancreas, the maximal volume is also decreased to <2 ml/kg body weight/h, but the enzyme activities are not greatly affected and the bicarbonate concentration even less so. Sometimes, normal responses are found temporarily after acute pancreatitis. Permanent sub-optimal responses are found in relapsing and progressive chronic pancreatitis. Acinar dysfunction and obstruction of the pancreatic duct produce differential effects with respect to volume, secretion rate, bicarbonate concentration and enzyme production. Simple stricture of the pancreatic duct results in a fall in volume. The bicarbonate concentration rises in patients with duodenal ulcer, cirrhosis of the liver, haemochromatosis and gall bladder disease following cholecystectomy.

Comment

CCK and PZ are now known to be the same compound. Steatorrhoea is a late feature of chronic pancreatic disease. This test is more complicated to perform than the 'Lundh test'.

SWEAT TEST[12]

Principle

In patients with cystic fibrosis (CF) there is impaired reabsorption of sodium and chloride in the ducts of the sweat glands. This results in high concentrations of these ions in the sweat, measurements of which constitute an important diagnostic parameter for this condition.

Indication

This test is used for confirming the diagnosis of clinically suspected CF, particularly in children, but also in adults.

Patient Preparation

No special preparation is required. This investigation may be performed on an in-patient or out-patient basis. Relatives should be warned that the test is uncomfortable, but usually not painful; an area of temporary skin erythema will result.

Protocol

This is a highly specialised procedure, based on the original procedure by L.E. Gibson and R.E. Cooke, but involving measurements of sweat sodium as well as of chloride. Chloride measurements are particularly useful in patients in whom the sweat sodium levels are equivocal (see below) and also where the amount of sweat obtained is <30 mg. The sweat test should only be performed by those carrying out the test regularly and who are in possession of the precise details of the protocol. The basic principles are as follows. The skin of both forearms is cleaned with de-ionised water on the extensor and flexor surfaces, preferably over areas of soft and fatty tissue. Special thick padded electrodes are attached firmly to the skin following pilocarpine (0.2%) application to the positive electrode/flexor surface and magnesium sulphate (0.1 M) to the negative electrode/ extensor surface. The current is passed, being gradually increased to 4 mA for 5 min and then gradually decreased, to each arm in turn. Carefully weighed filter papers (Whatman No. 41, tested for low sodium content) are then placed with forceps on the skin and covered with waterproof sealed polythene wrappings; they are applied to both arms. The filter papers are weighed again

134

30 min later in the laboratory (see below 'Sample Handling'). Up to 100 mg sweat should be collected if possible. **Caution: there is a danger of electrical burns.**

Sample Handling

The filter papers are returned to sealed plastic boxes without finger contact, and sent to the laboratory immediately for weighing, extraction and estimation of sodium and chloride.

Normal Response

In normal subjects the sweat sodium is <60 mmol/L, being much lower in infants; the chloride concentration is slightly less.

Interpretation

In patients with CF, the sweat sodium is >70 mmol/L, with the chloride concentration being slightly greater. Where levels of sodium lie in the range of 50–70 mmol/L, chloride estimation is particularly useful, not only as an aid to quality control, but also to provide information regarding the ratio of sodium/chloride. The sum of sodium and chloride, both being expressed in mmol/L, is also important; figures >140 mmol/L are suggestive of CF. If the sweat sample is <50 mg, patients with CF will have a sweat sodium concentration of >80 mmol/L; if the sweat sample is >250 mg this figure falls to >60 mmol/L. If positive, the test should be repeated a few weeks/months later in order to confirm the diagnosis of CF.

Comment

This is an important diagnostic test. Very great accuracy in sample weighing is necessary. Particular attention must be paid to avoiding contamination of the Whatman filter paper, which should be handled with forceps only, at all stages throughout the procedure.

TETRACOSACTRIN (SYNACTHEN, CORTROSYN) STIMULATION TEST
Five hour procedure

Principle
Tetracosactrin is a synthetic preparation comprising the first 24 amino acids of ACTH. It stimulates the normal adrenal cortex to produce cortisol, failure to respond indicating impaired adrenocortical function.

Indication
This test is indicated for confirming clinically strongly suspected primary adrenocortical insufficiency in patients in whom there is a doubtful response in the short 'Tetracosactrin (Synacthen, Cortrosyn) stimulation test', which is a screening procedure.

Patient Preparation
This test can be used as an in-patient or out-patient procedure. The patient is placed in a reclining position to rest for 30 min prior to the test. Smoking is not permitted. Pharmacological doses of glucocorticoids should not have been administered for the previous 12 h. **Caution: withdrawal of glucocorticoids may be dangerous.**

Protocol
This test is best commenced early in the morning. Base-line venous blood (5 ml) is collected into a plain glass bottle for serum cortisol, and a further 20 ml may be collected at the same time into a polythene bottle containing heparin, pre-cooled on ice, for plasma ACTH estimation (special collection, see Appendix III). Tetracosactrin Depot (1 mg) is injected intramuscularly. Venous blood (5 ml) is collected 1 h and 5 h later for serum cortisol estimation.

Sample Handling
This is as for serum cortisol and plasma ACTH estimation; the sample for ACTH estimation should be processed immediately.

Normal Response
The base-line serum cortisol should be >140 nmol/L. This should

136

rise at 1 h to between 600 and 1250 nmol/L and at 5 h to between 1000 and 1800 nmol/L. The base-line plasma ACTH should lie within the reference range of 10–80 ng/L.

Interpretation

A normal response excludes primary adrenocortical hypofunction, but does not exclude hypofunction secondary to pituitary disease or prolonged excessive glucocorticoid therapy. An impaired response suggests primary or secondary adrenocortical insufficiency, and these should be differentiated by using the prolonged 'Tetracosactrin (Synacthen, Cortrosyn) stimulation test'. A normal baseline plasma ACTH level excludes primary adrenocortical insufficiency.

Comment

Measurement of plasma ACTH at 11.00 pm, in addition, would provide information relating to diurnal variation and its loss. If the results of serum cortisol estimations are available quickly, and indicate an impaired response, the test may be extended to become part of the prolonged 'Tetracosactrin (Synacthen, Cortrosyn) stimulation test'.

137

TETRACOSACTRIN (SYNACTHEN, CORTROSYN) STIMULATION TEST
Prolonged procedure

Principle

Tetracosactrin is a synthetic preparation comprising the first 24 amino acids of ACTH. It stimulates the normal adrenal cortex to produce cortisol, failure to respond indicating impaired adrenocortical function.

Indication

This test is indicated in order to differentiate primary adrenocortical insufficiency, e.g. Addison's disease or following withdrawal of previous long-term high dose glucocorticoid drug therapy (including topical steroids), from insufficiency secondary to pituitary disease.

Patient Preparation

This is an in-patient procedure. The patient remains at rest in bed prior to collection of the base-line blood sample. Smoking is not permitted. Neither pharmacological nor routine replacement glucocorticoid drug therapy should have been given for the previous 12 h, or during the test. **Caution: with .:awal of glucocorticoids may be dangerous.** Dexamethasone (1 mg), which does not interfere with serum cortisol estimations, should be given orally each day as a precaution against developing an adrenocortical crisis.

Protocol

Base-line venous blood (5 ml) is collected into a plain glass bottle. Tetracosactrin Depot (1 mg) is administered intramuscularly daily at the same time for 3 days. Further blood samples are collected 5 h after each injection.

Sample Handling

This is as for serum cortisol estimation.

Normal Response

The base-line serum cortisol level should be >140 nmol/L with a rise

138

5 h following the first injection to at least 1000–1800 nmol/L, being maintained in excess of this level throughout the test.

Interpretation

No response at the end of 3 days confirms primary adrenocortical insufficiency. An impaired but increasing response indicates adrenocortical insufficiency secondary to pituitary disease or prolonged excessive glucocorticoid administration.

Comment

Sodium and water retention may lead to oedema and heart failure. Allergic reactions to tetracosactrin may occur, but are rare. This test is probably rendered unnecessary if base-line plasma ACTH assays are available.

TETRACOSACTRIN (SYNACTHEN, CORTROSYN) STIMULATION TEST
Short Procedure

Principle

Tetracosactrin is a synthetic preparation comprising the first 24 amino acids of ACTH. It stimulates the normal adrenal cortex to produce cortisol, failure to respond indicating impaired adrenocortical function.

Indication

This test is of value in patients with suspected primary adrenocortical insufficiency, e.g. Addison's disease, and also during the later stages of withdrawal and following total cessation of previous long-term high dose glucocorticoid drug therapy, including topical preparations. It is a screening test.

Patient Preparation

This test can be used either as an in-patient or out-patient screening procedure. The patient is placed in a reclining position to rest for 30 min prior to the test. Smoking is not permitted. Pharmacological doses of glucocorticoids should not have been administered for the previous 12 h. **Caution: withdrawal of glucocorticoids may be dangerous.**

Protocol

This test is best performed early in the morning. Base-line venous blood (5 ml) is collected into a plain glass bottle. Tetracosactrin (250 μg) is administered intramuscularly or intravenously and 30 min later a further blood sample is collected.

Sample Handling

This is as for serum cortisol estimation.

Normal Response

The base-line serum cortisol level should be >140 nmol/L. This should rise at 30 min to >550 nmol/L, with the rise being >200 nmol/L irrespective of the initial level.

140

Interpretation

Failure to meet the normal criteria indicates adrenocortical insufficiency due to any cause. Low normal levels and responses are compatible with some degree of adrenocortical impairment and are an indication for further investigation using the depot form of tetracosactrin, i.e. the five hour 'Tetracosactrin (Synacthen, Cortrosyn) stimulation test'. A clearly normal response excludes primary and secondary adrenocortical insufficiency and indicates that further tests are not required.

Comment

This investigation is frequently employed, being a safe, useful, and practical screening test. Allergic reactions to tetracosactrin are a possibility, but rarely occur. It is often used repeatedly in order to assess adrenocortical function during the later stages of slow withdrawal of prolonged, high dose, glucocorticoid therapy. It may also be used to confirm a previously made diagnosis of Addison's disease in patients receiving replacement therapy.

141

THIAZIDE CHALLENGE TEST

Principle

Administration of thiazide compounds causes inhibition of urinary calcium excretion. This may result in hypercalcaemia, not only in patients with autonomous parathyroid hormone (PTH) secretion, but also in those with other states of high calcium turnover.

Indication

This test is useful in patients with hypercalciuria, especially if normocalcaemic, for the purpose of differentiating idiopathic hypercalciuria from early hyperparathyroidism (primary, tertiary or ectopic) and from vitamin D intoxication.

Patient Preparation

The patient would probably have been receiving a low calcium diet as treatment for hypercalciuria, but should revert to normal calcium intake for the duration of this test.

Protocol

Hydrochlorothiazide (50 mg twice daily) is administered orally for 7–10 days. Venous blood (15 ml) is collected without stasis, using a polythene syringe, on 2 successive days prior to thiazide administration, into a plain glass bottle and a plain polythene bottle for estimation of serum calcium and PTH respectively (special collection, see Appendix III). Repeat blood samples are collected on the last 2 days of thiazide administration.

Sample Handling

This is as for serum calcium, albumin and PTH estimation, samples being sent to the laboratory immediately.

Normal Response

The serum calcium level, corrected for albumin, may rise by up to 0.38 mmol/L, usually remaining within or perhaps rising to just above the upper limit of the reference range; it should, however, remain at <2.75 mmol/L. The serum PTH should fall to undetectable levels.

142

Interpretation

Patients with primary, tertiary or ectopic hyperparathyroidism will develop hypercalcaemia, with serum calcium levels rising to >2.75 mmol/L (i.e. an unequivocally abnormal response) and accompanied by failure of suppression of serum PTH. Patients with idiopathic hypercalciuria may have a raised base-line level of serum PTH due to secondary hyperparathyroidism, but this will suppress in response to thiazide administration. Patients with vitamin D intoxication will develop hypercalcaemia in response to thiazide administration, but will have undetectable serum PTH levels throughout.

Comment

This test, being somewhat unpredictable and non-specific is not frequently used. Sometimes, urine collections for calcium excretion are advocated, but some fall in excretion is expected in all circumstances and interpretation on a quantitative basis is difficult. However, urine calcium measurement may be of value when used as an index of thiazide compliance. The diuretic effect of thiazide administration will result in large urine volumes.

THYROTROPHIN-RELEASING HORMONE (TRH) STIMULATION TEST
Intravenous procedure

Principle

Thyrotrophin-releasing hormone (TRH) is a hypothalamic tripeptide, synthesised by, stored within and released from the hypothalamus. It stimulates the synthesis and release of thyroid-stimulating hormone (TSH) and prolactin (PRL) from the anterior pituitary gland. In hyperthyroidism administration of exogenous TRH is characterised by impaired release of TSH, whereas in primary hypothyroidism there is exaggerated release; in both instances there is altered target organ feedback. In hypothalamic disorders the TSH response is delayed on account of time being required for its synthesis within the pituitary gland.

Indication

This test is indicated in several circumstances. The main indication is in clinically marginal hyperthyroidism, with equivocal serum thyroxine (T4) and tri-iodothyronine (T3) (total and free) levels. It is particularly useful in atypical hyperthyroid patients, presenting with either isolated eye signs (bilateral or unilateral), or atrial fibrillation, the latter sometimes being seen as a lone feature of hyperthyroidism, especially in the elderly. A further indication is in some cases of equivocal primary hypothyroidism, in which the serum TSH level, though still within, is close to the upper end of the reference range. In mild hypothyroidism, secondary to suspected hypopituitarism, TRH stimulation may also be used as part of the 'Hypothalamic-pituitary (anterior) function (combined hypothalamic-releasing hormone/insulin) test', and 'Pituitary (anterior) function (combined hypothalamic-releasing hormone/arginine vasopressin) test'. Finally, this test is indicated in patients with suspected hypothalamic disease.

Patient Preparation

No special preparation is essential, but ideally the patient should fast overnight and during the test, and be at rest. Smoking is not permitted.

Protocol

This test is best performed in the early morning and repeat tests (if required) should be carried out at the same time of day, but not within 7 days. Venous blood (5 ml) is collected into a plain glass bottle, following which an injection of TRH (200 μg) is given intravenously as a bolus. Further samples of blood are collected at 20 and 60 min.

Sample Handling

This is as for serum TSH and PRL estimation.

Normal Response

The base-line level of serum TSH should be <7 mIU/L, with a significant rise of >2 mIU/L (but with peak <25 mIU/L) at 20 min in response to TRH, and with a return towards the base-line value at 60 min.

Interpretation

In this test, a flat or nearly flat response (i.e. a serum TSH rise of <2 mIU/L) with a low base-line level occurs in hyperthyroidism, including the early stages of the disease. Early primary hypothyroidism displays a high base-line level together with an exaggerated response at 20 min. It is important to exclude hypofunction of the anterior pituitary gland whenever there is an impaired response; this may also occur in acromegaly, Cushing's syndrome, after adrenocortical steroid therapy and following previous thyroid therapy. A delayed peak occurs in hypothalamic disease, with the 60 min sample showing a higher level than the 20 min sample. An exaggerated response is seen in pregnancy and in patients receiving oral contraceptives. In cases of reduced end-organ sensitivity to circulating thyroid hormones, there may be an elevated response in this test. Normal elderly subjects show a smaller rise of serum TSH, but always >2 mIU/L. In patients with chronic renal failure or liver disease the serum TSH response to TRH is prolonged but delayed. Occasionally, apparently healthy subjects fail to respond. Drugs which modify the TSH response to TRH include antithyroid compounds, L-dopa, phenothiazines, metoclopramide, bromocriptine, salicylates and theophylline; T4 and T3 administration will affect the response

Comment

This is a very useful test when carried out by itself for confirming the diagnosis of hyperthyroidism when other tests are equivocal. It is not suitable for patients with bronchial asthma or myocardial ischaemia, in whom the oral 'Thyrotrophin-releasing hormone (TRH) stimulation test' is preferable.

THYROTROPHIN-RELEASING HORMONE (TRH) STIMULATION TEST
Oral procedure

Principle

Thyrotrophin-releasing hormone (TRH) is a hypothalamic tripeptide synthesised by, stored within and released from the hypothalamus. It stimulates the synthesis and release of thyroid-stimulating hormone (TSH) from the anterior pituitary gland. In hyperthyroidism administration of exogenous TRH is characterised by impaired release of TSH due to altered target organ feedback.

Indication

This test is useful in suspected hyperthyroidism in patients who also have bronchial asthma or myocardial ischaemia, for whom the intravenous 'Thyrotrophin-releasing hormone (TRH) stimulation test' is unsuitable.

Patient Preparation

The patient should fast overnight and for the duration of the test but is allowed to drink water. Smoking is not permitted.

Protocol

TRH (40 mg) is given orally in half a glass of water during the morning. Venous blood (5 ml) is collected at 0, 3, 5 and 8 h into plain glass bottles.

Sample Handling

This is as for serum TSH, thyroxine (T4) and tri-iodothyronine (T3) estimation.

Normal Response

The base-line level of serum TSH should be <7 mIU/L with the peak value being >5 mIU/L but <30 mIU/L in either the 3 or 5 h samples. The serum T3 concentration begins to rise at 3 h and the serum T4 concentration at 5 or 8 h. In the 8 h sample there is a return of serum TSH to the base-line level.

147

Interpretation

A flat serum TSH response occurs in patients with hyperthyroidism and also in some normal subjects. No significant change is seen in the base-line serum T3 and T4 values at 3, 5 or 8 h in hyperthyroidism. Drugs which modify the TSH response to TRH include anti-thyroid compounds, L-dopa, phenothiazines, metoclopramide, bromocriptine, salicylates and theophylline; T4 and T3 administration also affects the response.

Comment

In practice, this investigation is usually carried out in order to exclude hyperthyroidism by virtue of a normal response, rather than to confirm the diagnosis. This is because a flat response is obtained, not only in hyperthyroidism (and hypopituitarism), but also in some normal subjects. The incidence of a flat response in normal subjects is less than with the intravenous 'Thyrotrophin--releasing hormone (TRH) stimulation test'.

L-TRYPTOPHAN LOAD TEST

Principle
In vitamin B_6 (pyridoxal phosphate) deficiency, the normal conversion of L-tryptophan to nicotinic acid is impaired beyond 3-hydroxykynurenic acid; following conversion the latter is excreted in the urine as xanthurenic acid in larger amounts than normal, particularly following an L-tryptophan load.

Indication
This test is indicated in suspected vitamin B_6 deficiency.

Patient Preparation
The patient fasts overnight, but is encouraged to drink water freely in the early morning on the day on which the L-tryptophan load is administered, in order to facilitate adequate urine output.

Protocol
A 24 h urine collection is made into a bottle containing 2 ml toluene, prior to administration of an oral dose of L-tryptophan (2 g) dissolved in water, for determination of xanthurenic acid (special collection, see Appendix III). A further 24 h urine collection is then made. Normal meals may be taken commencing 2 h after the L-tryptophan load.

Sample Handling
Each sample of urine is sent separately to the laboratory without delay and stored at +4 °C for estimation of xanthurenic acid.

Normal Response
The normal excretion of xanthurenic acid is <50 mg/24 h.

Interpretation
The 24 h urinary excretion of xanthurenic acid is increased 2- to 10-fold in vitamin B_6 deficiency, although this cannot be regarded as specific. Increased excretion is also associated with the taking of oral contraceptive preparations.

149

L-Tryptophan load test

Comment

This is a useful and safe test. It is more satisfactory and easier to perform than making direct measurements of vitamin B_6 in the blood. L-Tryptophan may cause nausea, drowsiness and headache. Normalisation of xanthurenic acid excretion is expected following vitamin B_6 therapy in cases of deficiency.

VITAMIN A ABSORPTION TEST

Principle

Oral administration of the fat-soluble vitamin A, followed by its estimation in serum, provides an index of the fat absorptive capacity of the small intestine.

Indication

This is a screening test for intestinal malabsorption syndromes.

Patient Preparation

Liquid paraffin medication should be avoided for 3 days prior to the test. The patient fasts overnight, but a normal diet may be resumed 2 h after the test dose of vitamin A has been taken. Smoking is not permitted.

Protocol

Vitamin A palmitate (7500 IU/kg body weight, maximum 350 000 IU) is administered orally in oil with a light meal. Venous blood (10 ml) is collected into a plain glass bottle prior to giving the test dose, and again at 4, 5 and 6 h for serum vitamin A determination (special collection, see Appendix III).

Sample Handling

Blood specimens must be protected from light, at and from the moment of collection, and dispatched to the laboratory for serum vitamin A estimation immediately.

Normal Response

The base-line serum vitamin A level is 1.0–2.3 μmol/L, rising after the vitamin A load to 7–21 μmol/L in any or all of the 3 samples.

Interpretation

A low base-line serum vitamin A concentration with a flat or delayed peak following the vitamin A load is suggestive of malabsorption.

151

Comment

The test is of limited value, as other tests are necessary for confirmation; it is only occasionally performed. It does not differentiate pancreatic disease from other malabsorption syndromes; the test is also abnormal in hepatocellular disease and in hypothyroidism. The carotene absorption test is similar in principle but is less satisfactory in that it requires 3 days for completion and is regarded as obsolete.

VITAMIN B$_{12}$ ABSORPTION (DICOPAC, Amersham International plc) TEST[13]

Principle

In pernicious anaemia there is defective absorption of vitamin B$_{12}$ (cyanocobalamin) caused by the absence of intrinsic factor (IF) in the stomach. This defect can be quantified, following oral administration of radioactively labelled vitamin B$_{12}$, the low absorption of which is corrected by concomitant administration of IF. The loading dose of parenteral non-radioactive vitamin B$_{12}$, given prior to and/or at the start of the test, is for the purpose of saturating the vitamin B$_{12}$ binding sites, thus ensuring that any radioactivity absorbed is readily excreted and not taken up by the tissues. Measurement of urinary radioactivity is used as the index of absorption of the isotope, assuming renal glomerular function to be normal. Vitamin B$_{12}$ absorption may also be affected in generalised intestinal malabsorption.

Indication

This test helps in the suspected diagnosis of pernicious anaemia (Addisonian anaemia) and also provides evidence for the diagnosis of generalised malabsorption.

Patient Preparation

The patient fasts overnight and for 2 h following administration of the test dose. The patient should not have received other radioactive isotopes in the recent past. The test may be performed on in-patients or out-patients.

Protocol

One capsule each of ^{58}Co-vitamin B$_{12}$ (0.25 μg; 29.6 kBq, 0.8 μCi) and ^{57}Co-vitamin B$_{12}$ (0.25 μg; 18.5 kBq, 0.5 μCi), the latter being bound to human gastric juice, is administered orally at the same time, together with non-radioactive vitamin B$_{12}$ (1000 μg) intramuscularly. Immediately beforehand, the bladder is emptied and the urine discarded; a 24 h urine collection is commenced into a plain polythene bottle.

153

Sample Handling

The 24 h urine sample is sent to the laboratory where both ^{57}Co and ^{58}Co are measured in the urine, together with the urine volume, in order to assess both the total excretion and the ratio between the 2 isotopes.

Normal Response

The reference range for either isotope is excretion in the first 24 h of 10–20% of the dose administered, with a ^{57}Co/^{58}Co ratio of 0.8–1.3.

Interpretation

The urine of patients with pernicious anaemia contains 5–14% ^{57}Co and 0.5–5.0% ^{58}Co, in the first 24 h after administration of the dose, with a ^{57}Co/^{58}Co ratio of 1.8–15.0. The urine of patients with generalised intestinal malabsorption contains <4% of either isotope, with a normal ^{57}Co/^{58}Co ratio. The ratio is particularly important when urine collection is incomplete, or in the presence of renal impairment.

Comment

This commercial kit is designed to give maximum information about vitamin B$_{12}$ absorption, with involvement of minimum specimen collection, on account of combining both Part I and II of the 'Vitamin B$_{12}$ absorption (Schilling) test'. It overcomes the difficulty of obtaining IF suitable for administration to humans as a separate entity. The sensitivity of the test is less than that of the traditional 'Schilling test', where Parts I and II are performed separately. Occasionally, this test may be used to exclude pernicious anaemia as a cause of undiagnosed vitamin B$_{12}$ deficiency, e.g due either to diet or to a defect of the ileal mucosal cell receptors for vitamin B$_{12}$. An alternative test is the 'Vitamin B$_{12}$ absorption (Schilling) test'.

VITAMIN B$_{12}$ ABSORPTION (SCHILLING) TEST

Principle

In pernicious anaemia there is defective absorption of vitamin B$_{12}$ (cyanocobalamin) caused by the absence of intrinsic factor (IF) in the stomach. This defect can be quantified following oral administration of radioactively labelled vitamin B$_{12}$, the low absorption of which is corrected by concomitant administration of IF. The loading dose of parenteral non-radioactive vitamin B$_{12}$, given prior to and/or at the start of the test, is for the purpose of saturating the vitamin B$_{12}$ binding sites, thus ensuring that any radioactivity absorbed is readily excreted and not taken up by the tissues. Measurement of urinary radioactivity is used as the index of absorption of the isotope, assuming renal glomerular function to be normal. Vitamin B$_{12}$ absorption may also be affected in generalised intestinal malabsorption.

Indication

This test is of value in establishing the diagnosis of pernicious anaemia (Addisonian anaemia), whether or not treatment with vitamin B$_{12}$ has already commenced. In addition, the test can provide contributory evidence for the diagnosis of generalised malabsorption.

Patient Preparation

The patient fasts overnight and for 2 h following administration of the test dose. The patient should not have received other radioactive isotopes in the recent past. The test may be performed on in-patients or out-patients.

Protocol

Part I of the 'Vitamin B$_{12}$ absorption (Schilling) test' involves administration of non-radioactive vitamin B$_{12}$ (1000 μg) intramuscularly, followed immediately by ^{58}Co-vitamin B$_{12}$ (0.5 μg approximately; 18.5 kBq, 0.5 μCi) given orally in 50 ml of water; the rinsings from the container are also taken, in order to ensure that the dose is complete. Part II of the 'Schilling test' can be performed 72 h later and consists of repeating Part I with, in addition, administration of one capsule of IF (Amersham International plc). Immediately before

155

commencing either part of the test, the bladder is emptied and the urine discarded; a 24 h urine collection in a plain polythene bottle is started at this time.

Sample Handling

The 24 h urine collection is sent to the laboratory for measurement of urine volume and radioactivity.

Normal Response

Normally >10% of the administered dose should be excreted in the first 24 h in Part 1 of the test, with no significant increase in Part II.

Interpretation

In Part I of the test, excretion of <1.5% of the administered ^{58}Co is diagnostic of pernicious anaemia; this is assuming that the patient took the dose, that there was no vomiting and that urine collection was complete. Excretion of 4–8% is compatible with generalised intestinal malabsorption. Impaired glomerular filtration delays excretion and produces a spuriously low result in the first 24 h collection, but further collections over the next few days would permit summation of radioactivity excreted over that period; in these circumstances a total value of >10% excretion of ^{58}Co would indicate normal vitamin B$_{12}$ absorption. Administration of other radioactive isotopes to the patient will produce spuriously high values of radioactivity, though these may decay rapidly, unlike the radioactive cobalt isotopes used here; repeat counting of the samples 1 week later may, therefore, be informative. In Part II of the test there is, in patients with pernicious anaemia, correction by IF of the low ^{58}Co excretion found in Part I of the test. There will, however, be no effect on the intermediate values found in generalised malabsorption.

Comment

A Part III of the 'Schilling test' is available, in which there is administration for 5 days of a gastrointestinally active antibiotic, prior to repeat of the Part II test. If this procedure corrects an intermediate response in Part II, this suggests that the basis for the malabsorption lies in bacterial consumption of the vitamin B$_{12}$, e.g. a blind loop syndrome or the presence of organisms within intestinal diverticulae. Part III of the test is, however, rarely used. Part I of the 'Schilling test', even without Part II, is an extremely good test for pernicious anaemia, even when vitamin B$_{12}$ therapy has commenced; indeed, it is essential that vitamin B$_{12}$ binding sites be saturated by intramuscular vitamin B$_{12}$ before the oral isotope is given. Occasionally, this test may be used to exclude pernicious anaemia as a cause of undiagnosed vitamin B$_{12}$ deficiency, e.g. due either to diet or to a defect of the ileal mucosal cell receptors for vitamin B$_{12}$. An alternative test is the 'Vitamin B$_{12}$ absorption (Dicopac, Amersham International plc) test'.

157

VITAMIN C SATURATION TEST

Principle
Administration of a standard dose of vitamin C (ascorbic acid) to patients suffering from gross deficiency of this vitamin leads to rapid uptake by the depleted tissues, with the result that none is available for excretion in the urine.

Indication
The test is useful in patients suspected of having vitamin C deficiency on account of malnutrition (often being in association with other confirmed vitamin deficiencies), or when there is clinical evidence of frank scurvy.

Patient Preparation
Neither therapeutic vitamin preparations nor foods containing vitamin C must be given either prior to, or during the test. Water intake, however, is to be encouraged, in order to facilitate urine collection.

Protocol
Vitamin C (11 mg/kg of body weight) is given orally at 9.00 am; the bladder is emptied at 1.00 pm and the urine discarded. Urine is collected between 1.00 and 3.00 pm into a dark bottle containing 20 ml of glacial acetic acid for vitamin C estimation (special collection, see Appendix III). The test is repeated on the following and subsequent days.

Sample Handling
The urine specimens must be sent immediately to the laboratory and estimated as soon as possible for vitamin C.

Normal Response
At least 50 mg of vitamin C should appear in the urine on the first or second day.

Interpretation
In moderate or severe vitamin C deficiency, with this test repeated

158

daily, it may take from 1-3 weeks for vitamin C to appear in the urine.

Comment

This is a useful but not commonly employed procedure, which may be used when leucocyte vitamin C measurements cannot be undertaken. Leucocyte vitamin C content is a better guide to body vitamin C stores; the test is, however, difficult to perform and is not always readily available.

WATER DEPRIVATION TEST

Principle

In patients with polyuria, the response of both urine osmolality and output to water deprivation differentiates conditions of overhydration from diabetes insipidus, as long as osmotic diuresis and chronic renal failure have been excluded.

Indication

The test is useful for the assessment of patients with polyuria suspected of having water intoxication (including iatrogenic intoxication and psychogenic polydipsia) or diabetes insipidus of hypothalamic, posterior pituitary or nephrogenic origin. Diabetes mellitus, other causes of osmotic diuresis and renal failure must previously have been excluded. **Caution: pre-renal uraemia is a hazard in patients with renal impairment.**

Patient Preparation

The patient fasts overnight and during the procedure, but free access to fluids should be allowed prior to the test. The patient should rest in bed. Smoking is not permitted.

Protocol

The patient should pass urine in the early morning with suprapubic pressure, in order to ensure complete emptying of the bladder; the urine is saved. Venous blood (5 ml) should be collected at approximately 9.00 am into a plain glass bottle. A urine aliquot is also collected at this time into a plain glass bottle. The patient now commences the phase of complete fluid deprivation and is weighed accurately at this point. Blood and urine samples are repeated later in the day and, if necessary, again the following day until the serum osmolality rises to >295 mmol/kg; however, measurements need not normally continue for more than 48 h. The patient should be weighed again during, and at the end of, the test. Patients with suspected psychogenic polydipsia should be observed closely throughout the test to prevent surreptitious water intake.

Sample Handling

Blood and urine should be handled as for electrolyte assays, estimation being made of serum and urine osmolality, serum sodium and urine volume.

Normal Response

The serum osmolality should not rise to >295 mmol/kg at any time, but the urine osmolality should rise rapidly towards 800 mmol/kg, accompanied by a marked fall in volume. The serum sodium concentration should not rise to >144 mmol/L, and the patient should not lose >3% body weight at maximum.

Interpretation

A high base-line serum osmolality, rising rapidly during the test, together with failure to develop an appropriate rise in urine osmolality, and accompanied by persisting high urine volumes, indicates diabetes insipidus of hypothalamic, posterior pituitary or nephrogenic origin. Patients with hypothalamic diabetes insipidus (including those with neurosurgical damage, particularly following removal of a craniopharyngioma) will, in addition, develop significant hypernatraemia and may characteristically show decreased or absent thirst. Patients with diabetes insipidus of posterior pituitary origin may exhibit rapid loss of up to 3% of body weight and become unwell at which point the test must be discontinued; patients will exhibit very severe thirst. Patients with iatrogenic water intoxication (e.g. inappropriate intravenous fluid therapy) will show a normal but delayed response. Patients with psychogenic polydipsia will also show a normal response; however, due to the chronic nature of the condition, there may be some impairment of ability to concentrate the urine, resulting in a less than optimal rise in urine osmolality. Patients with polyuria due to chronic renal failure would display high serum osmolality on account of mild dehydration, in addition to the elevated serum urea; the serum osmolality would continue to rise further during the test with little change in urine osmolality. However, water deprivation should not be performed in patients with known renal failure, and such patients should be excluded from this procedure.

161

Comment

This test is best performed with frequent monitoring of serum and urine changes in response to water deprivation, rather than adhering to fixed time regimens. It should be noted that temporary diabetes insipidus may follow craniotomy or head injury. This test should be considered together with the 'Desmopressin acetate (1-deamino-8-D-arginine vasopressin, DDAVP) response test'.

WATER LOAD TEST

Principle

Ability to excrete a standard oral water load, as assessed by measurement of urine volume, together with estimation of serum and urine osmolality and serum sodium, is dependent upon normal hepatic, renal, adrenocortical, pituitary and hypothalamic function.

Indication

The main indication for this test is in the assessment of hypothalamic function, though the procedure may also be used as a means of indirectly assessing function of the other systems, as indicated above.

Patient Preparation

The patient should be free from stress and pain. Smoking is not permitted. Sodium intake should not have been excessive during the previous 48 h.

Protocol

The bladder is emptied completely at approximately 9.00 am, the urine being saved. Venous blood (5 ml) should be collected at this time. Water (1 L) is then administered by mouth over a period of 10 min. Urine is collected at hourly intervals for 5 h and a further blood sample is collected at 5 h.

Sample Handling

Blood and urine are processed as for electrolyte and osmolality assays, estimation being made of serum osmolality and sodium, and urine osmolality and volume.

Normal Response

The serum osmolality should not fall to <278 mmol/kg and the urine osmolality should fall rapidly to <200 mmol/kg. The urine volume should rise to enable excretion, in the first 5 h, of 80% of the water load. The serum sodium concentration should not fall to <132 mmol/L.

163

Interpretation

Failure to excrete a water load, characterised by absence of fall in urine osmolality and absence of rise in urine volume, is a feature of adrenocortical insufficiency, hypothalamic damage with loss of osmoreceptors (including patients with neurosurgical damage, particularly following removal of a craniopharyngioma), chronic hepatic disease, renal failure and inappropriate secretion of vasopressin (syndrome of inappropriate ADH secretion, SIADH). Patients with intestinal malabsorption syndromes and congestive cardiac failure also exhibit failure of the normal response to a water load.

Comment

The test is, in fact, contraindicated in the presence of congestive cardiac failure. It may be dangerous, also, in patients with inappropriate secretion of vasopressin, in whom direct measurement of plasma and urine ADH may be helpful and safer, though rarely necessary and often unavailable. In hypothalamic damage with loss of osmoreceptor control, useful information may be obtained by the very careful monitoring of serum and urine osmolality following cautious administration of the fluid load; this provides a means of assessing loss of osmolality control. Moreover, hyponatraemia is easily induced in these patients, who previously exhibited hypernatraemia associated with dehydration; this is due to relative 'fixity' of urine osmolality, despite wide variation in fluid intake and excretion.

WHISKY STIMULATION TEST

Principle

Ethyl alcohol ingestion (in the form of whisky) stimulates the release of calcitonin (CT) from certain tumours, especially medullary carcinoma of the thyroid gland (MCT).

Indication

This is the basis of a screening test for suspected MCT.

Patient Preparation

The patient fasts overnight and remains at rest in bed for the duration of the test. Smoking is not permitted.

Protocol

Whisky (50 ml) is given by mouth over a few minutes. Venous blood (15 ml) is collected in a pre-cooled polythene syringe at 0, 3, 10, 15 and 30 min for plasma CT estimation (special collection, see Appendix III).

Sample Handing

Blood is transferred immediately to a polythene bottle containing heparin, pre-cooled with ice. The specimens must be sent to the laboratory immediately. Visible haemolysis invalidates the results.

Normal Response

The plasma CT should be <100 ng/L in all specimens in males, and <50 ng/L in females.

Interpretation

Following whisky administration, there is a marked rise in plasma CT in patients with MCT, often associated with flushing and diarrhoea.

Comment

This is a relatively pleasant and effective test, though flushing and diarrhoea may occur as side effects in patients with a positive response. Whisky is only one of several factors known to increase CT release; others include calcium and pentagastrin.

165

D-XYLOSE ABSORPTION TEST

Principle

D-Xylose, a non-metabolised monosaccharide (a pentose), is estimated in the urine following oral administration. It acts as a marker for assessing carbohydrate absorption and serves as a measure of generalised intestinal malabsorption of non-pancreatic origin.

Indication

This test is a screening procedure used in the differential diagnosis of malabsorption syndromes (including coeliac disease and tropical sprue) from steatorrhoea of pancreatic origin.

Patient Preparation

The patient fasts overnight but is encouraged to drink water freely in the early morning on the day of the test. There must be no eating during the test. Smoking is not permitted.

Protocol

The bladder is emptied completely and the urine discarded. D-Xylose (5 g) dissolved in 250 ml of water, is administered orally over a few minutes, followed by a further 250 ml of water in order to ensure adequate urine output. Urine is collected for the next 5 h into a dark bottle. Venous blood (5 ml) is collected at 2 h into a plain glass bottle.

Sample Handing

The urine is sent to the laboratory as soon as the collection is complete; the blood sample is also sent without delay following collection. Estimation is made of serum and urine D-xylose, and of urine volume.

Normal Response

There should be excretion of >8.0 mmol/5h (>1.2 g/5h) of D-xylose in the urine; the serum concentration of D-xylose should be >1.33 mmol/L.

Interpretation

In the presence of coeliac disease, tropical sprue and other non-pancreatic malabsorption syndromes, there is both decreased urinary D-xylose excretion and low serum D-xylose concentration. Renal glomerular disease, even in the presence of normal intestinal absorption, may result in delayed excretion, and hence low urine D-xylose output in the 5 h period, but in this circumstance there is a normal or high serum D-xylose level. Low amounts in the urine and serum may be caused by failure of the patient to comply, vomiting of the dose or by delayed gastric emptying, especially in children. Low urine volumes of less than 100 ml in 5 h may also lead to unreliable results. In malabsorption of exocrine pancreatic origin, the result of this test is normal.

Comment

The test based on a 25 g dose of oral D-xylose is less frequently used nowadays. Diarrhoea and vomiting may be complications of this test, especially with the 25 g load, but these also feature in the 5 g load test, especially in children with coeliac disease.This test may be used serially in assessment of the response to a low gluten diet in patients with coeliac disease but is now being used less frequently with the more ready availability of jejunal biopsy.

ZINC TOLERANCE TEST

Principle

Administration of a standard oral dose of a readily absorbable inorganic zinc salt enables differentiation between zinc deficient and normal subjects. Assessment is based on observing the change in serum zinc level, particularly at 2 h after the dose, and also on measuring urinary excretion of zinc.

Indication

The test is useful in patients with suspected depletion of zinc, despite serum zinc levels being within the reference range.

Patient Preparation

The patient fasts overnight. Care should be taken to ensure that neither zinc-containing medications (including zinc insulin preparations), nor topical application of zinc ointments/creams are being prescribed.

Protocol

Zinc sulphate (200 mg, equivalent to 50 mg zinc) is administered orally in a small quantity of water followed by 2 rinses of the cup, in order to ensure that the full amount has been ingested. Venous blood (10ml) is collected using polythene syringes and stainless steel needles (not rubber containing vacuum tubes). Haemolysis invalidates the results. Blood samples are taken at 0, 2, 4 and 6 h for serum zinc determination (special collection, see Appendix III). A 24 h urine collection is made both before and after the zinc ingestion for urine zinc determination (special collection, see Appendix III).

Sample Handling

The serum is estimated for zinc concentration and the urine for both volume and zinc concentration.

Normal Response

A rise in serum zinc concentration of 50–100% occurs at 2 h and there should be an increased 24 h urinary excretion of zinc.

Interpretation

A rise in the serum zinc concentration at 2 h of less than 35%, with no change in urinary excretion, indicates body depletion of zinc despite base-line serum zinc concentration being within the accepted reference range; this is presuming that the patient complied, did not vomit shortly after receiving the dose, and had no delay in gastric emptying. Depletion of zinc may occur in neoplastic conditions (especially carcinoma of the bronchus), following burns and in elderly patients with leg ulcers. Gross deficiency is associated with long term zinc deficient parenteral feeding, especially in infancy; it also occurs in acrodermatitis enteropathica. Defective wound healing is a clinical feature of tissue zinc deficiency.

Comment

This is a newly described test which has yet to be fully evaluated. It supplements other tests for zinc deficiency, including zinc analysis of head hair.

APPENDIX I
PREPARATION OF THE PATIENT AND PATIENT AFTER-CARE

PREPARATION OF THE PATIENT

Many investigations require preparation of the patient beforehand, usually only for 12–15 hours, but in some instances preparation in the form of a special diet may be necessary several days in advance. It is particularly important to pay careful attention to the precise instructions with respect, for example, to 'fasting', 'fluids only', 'fluid restriction', 'nil by mouth', etc. and particularly to 'basal conditions'. Generally speaking, unless there are instructions to the contrary, the patient should be quietly at rest in bed having emptied the bladder at least one hour before the test begins and the patient should wear loose clothing to allow easy access to the arms for the purpose of collecting blood. Occasionally, exercise forms part of the test, but if so, specific instructions to that effect will be given. As a routine, smoking is not permitted. Tests should be carried out in the early morning, and oral medications continued, unless there are alternative specific instructions.

Fasting

This refers to the patient taking no food for a period of 8–15 hours prior to commencement of a test. No meals or drinks, with the exception of water, should be taken after 10.00 pm on the previous evening for a test commencing in the early morning. Water, up to 1 L, is allowed and indeed should be encouraged in order to facilitate urine collection, should this be necessary. Intravenous fluids may continue to be administered provided that they do not contain calories. There must be no nasogastric feeding. The patient's medicines and tablets should be continued. It should be noted that some medicines, particularly those prepared for children, may contain sugar.

Non-fasting

Occasionally, investigations require that the patient maintains a normal food intake, having a normal breakfast with respect to both solid food and fluid intake, together with

171

medicines and tablets. The patient should be prepared for the test, having been warned in advance that blood will be taken.

Prolonged fasting

For this, the patient is given neither food, nor calorie-containing infusions, perhaps for up to 72 hours. Smoking is not permitted throughout the whole of this period. 'Prolonged fasting' may need to be accompanied by the taking of exercise, within the capacity of the cardiac and respiratory systems. Clinical observation is necessary throughout.

Fluids only, fluid restriction and fluid loading.

In these situations water and fluids (which may contain calories and/or vitamins) are given by mouth, but all solid food is excluded. 'Fluids only' may be required in hospital practice in various situations, but is an unusual requirement for biochemical tests. In contrast, if specific instructions are given for biochemical tests with respect to 'fluid restriction' or 'fluid loading', the precise amount to be given must be stipulated, this generally relating to 'water only'.

Nil by mouth

This requires that the patient be given no solid food, no calorie-containing fluids and no water. Medication should be continued by mouth or parenterally, as should intravenous fluids, though if these contain calories this must be noted. It is particularly important to differentiate between 'fasting', as defined above, and 'nil by mouth'. The latter is, however, likely to result in some difficulties in urine collection; moreover, this instruction is unusual for biochemical tests, unlike the fasting state which is commonly required.

Basal conditions

The patient should be comfortable, recumbent in bed, clad in loose clothing with access available to the arms for venepuncture and at complete physical and mental rest. The ambient temperature should be favourable, the surroundings quiet, and the patient should have 'nil by mouth'. Smoking is not permitted. As a general rule, tests should be carried out in the early morning. Under special circumstances, e.g. for a basal metabolic rate (BMR) test, a single room is preferable; if not possible, curtains should be drawn around the bed. Ideally, patients for investigations requiring 'basal conditions' should be on a metabolic ward. The bladder should have been emptied at least one hour prior to commencement of the investigation and the urine discarded. If blood is to be collected, an intravenous catheter should be inserted at least half an hour prior to the start of the test.

Diet

Special diets such as 'high carbohydrate', 'low carbohydrate', or 'high protein', may need to be instituted several days prior to investigation.

Most of the above instructions apply to in-patients, but many may be used for out-patients also, though clearly in this situation, 'basal conditions', are not possible. Occasionally, however, it may be permissible to admit a patient for a period of several hours bed rest prior to investigation requiring 'basal conditions', but this is not ideal. Posture, though affecting the blood levels of some constituents, is not important unless stipulated; there are, however, some exceptions in which case specific details will be given.

PATIENT AFTER-CARE

It is important in the case of out-patients that the consequences of any investigations be anticipated. This applies particularly to hypotension, hypoglycaemia, or collapse, which may be precipitated by stress (e.g. anaesthesia or surgery) when adrenal or pituitary insufficiency has been suspected and recently investigated with reference to the testing of reserve function. Respiratory weakness may also be a danger in patients with periodic paralysis and myasthenia gravis. There may be haematological consequences following drug administration, such as platelet count reduction and this may not become apparent for some time. Attention should be given to the question of driving, particularly where drowsiness or confusion may arise following medication or investigation; in these circumstances, an out-patient should always be accompanied home.

APPENDIX II
SPECIMEN COLLECTION, HANDLING AND TRANSPORTATION – GENERAL PRINCIPLES

SPECIMEN COLLECTION

BLOOD

Venous blood

For most tests venous blood is required in amounts stipulated by the local laboratory; it should be collected with minimum stasis from a large vein, preferably the antecubital vein, the overlying skin having previously been cleaned and allowed to dry. A syringe or vacuum tube with a sharp, but not fine bore, needle is used. Blood is placed immediately, but slowly and gently and without rapid discharge, into the required series of bottles up to the mark indicated on each. These are labelled with name, time, date and hospital number. Checks should already have been made regarding possible risks, including hepatitis B, tendency of the patient to have fainting attacks and sensitivity to elastoplast. Specimens from known HIV-positive and AIDS patients and from those with hepatitis B, should be processed with particular precautions, both with respect to specimen handling and laboratory procedures. Where the bottle contains anticoagulants, there should be gentle inversion several times without delay – but the bottles should not be shaken. Blood should not be withdrawn from a limb into which an intravenous infusion is running. Unreliable results will occur if blood is taken soon after exchange transfusion, plasma exchange transfusion, intralipid infusion, or massive whole blood transfusion. Generally, the patient should be sitting or lying but, if in the former position, should be carefully observed for signs of impending syncope, especially if fasting. Once collected, blood must never be transferred from one bottle to another. Where large volumes or multiple samples are involved, the use of an intravenous catheter is recommended; this should be inserted 30 minutes prior to collection of the first sample,

175

particularly when anxiety is likely to affect the biochemical parameter being measured. If venous stasis has been necessary in order to obtain the samples, this should be documented, as also should anxiety, especially when blood has been taken for the first time or for certain specific tests, including serum prolactin (PRL), growth hormone (GH) and cortisol. In cases of difficulty, blood may be obtained from the femoral vein below the inguinal ligament and medial to the femoral artery, though this must be taken by a medical practitioner. If blood is being collected for cryoglobulins, the syringe and tubes must be pre-warmed to 37 °C and the specimen taken immediately to the laboratory in a warmed container to prevent precipitation of the protein.

Capillary blood

This is particularly suitable for glucose analysis and may be taken from the lateral border of the finger, lobe of the ear or, in the case of children, the heel. It is essential to obtain an adequate sample of blood without the application of local pressure.

Arterial blood

Collection of arterial blood is a more dangerous and painful procedure; it is taken by a medical practitioner, a local anaesthetic being used. If collection is for blood gas analysis, holding the breath or over-breathing should be avoided, as both will have a rapid effect on P_{CO_2} values.

Arterialised venous blood

Strictly speaking, 'arterialised venous blood' is a misnomer and refers to venous blood in a situation of local hyperaemia created by application of heat; it goes some way to becoming a substitute for proper arterial blood under certain circumstances, e.g. for blood gas analysis in children.

URINE

Random urine specimen

For many purposes all that is required is collection of approximately 20 ml of a freshly passed specimen of urine. This is made at any time, except for the first sample in the morning, into a plastic container without addition of preservative. This is different from a mid-stream specimen (MSU) which is required for microbiological purposes and which needs to be collected by a sterile procedure.

Early morning urine specimen

An early morning specimen is similar to a random urine collection, but merely consists of part of the first voidance of urine in the morning. If the whole specimen is required, specific instructions to this effect should be given.

24 hour urine collection

A polythene bottle of at least 2.5 L capacity, with a wide neck and a properly fitting stopper, should be supplied, together with a polythene funnel for females. The bottle may have to be specially prepared with regard to added acid or preservative and the label should indicate hazards associated with these. The bottle must, in other respects also, be fully labelled and issued with instructions as to how the urine collection is to be made. Female patients must be advised not to collect during menstruation. It is usually convenient for the collection to take place between, say, 8.00 am on the first day and 8.00 am on the following day, though it must be stressed that in order to fit in with other investigations the time of commencement and completion of the collection may vary, provided a full 24 hour sample is collected. At the start, the patient should empty the bladder completely, preferably standing in the case of men and using suprapubic pressure, the time being noted exactly and the urine discarded. The whole of each subsequent specimen is collected every time that urine is passed, up to and including the same time the following day, when the final specimen is placed in the bottle.

Patients should be advised not to pass urine shortly before the end of the 24 hour period, as it may then be difficult to pass urine again at the precise time of completion. If, for any reason, it is not possible to pass the last specimen at the precise time, the exact time at which it is passed should be noted, so that the laboratory is aware that the sample is, for instance, a 24.5 hour sample instead of a 24 hour sample; for many purposes this may be satisfactory, provided the information is supplied. The patient must be told to keep the stopper on the bottle at all times between sample collections and never to place it anywhere except back on the bottle, i.e. it should never be placed on a bench or floor because this could result in contamination; this would be particularly important for trace metal analysis. The same care needs to be taken with the polythene funnel when used for urinary collection by females.

If a second 24 hour sample is required (as is often the case), this can be commenced immediately following the first; urine is then placed in a second bottle until the second 24 hour period has been completed. For out-patients, the timing of the collection should be arranged so that specimens are not left around unnecessarily long before being sent to the laboratory; but, in any case, the bottle and its contents should be kept in a cool place.

From the point of view of the laboratory, a high degree of suspicion as to the correctness of a collection is aroused when presented with a bottle of urine just full to the brim, or when the urine volume is very low. Clearly, some patients will require 2 bottles for a single 24 hour urine collection. Patients must be instructed that when passing stools the urine should be collected separately.

On the ward, it must be emphasised that if part of a sample is lost, either by the patient or staff, the collection should be continued, but the loss clearly documented. Care must obviously be taken that contamination from other patient's urine does not occur; nevertheless, experience shows that this is perhaps more frequent than is generally realised.

In all instances, the entire specimen must be brought to the laboratory as soon as possible. If analyses are to be carried out elsewhere or at a later date, it may suffice for the laboratory to retain an aliquot taken after adequate mixing, the 24 hour urine volume being noted.

Timed urine samples other than 24 hour collections

On occasions, timed samples (usually of the order of 1–6 hours) are required, in which case the same principles apply as in the collection of 24 hour specimens, except that smaller bottles are provided and very accurate timing is necessary. This is particularly important for, say, 2 consecutive urine collections as required in some clearance tests, with timed blood samples being taken approximately halfway through each period. In these circumstances it is important that the patient be well hydrated prior to the test and that this state be maintained throughout, in order to be able to pass urine in reasonable quantities when requested to do so and, as far as possible, to produce equal amounts in equal periods of time. Nevertheless, quite apart from clearance tests, the patient may, for example, be given a series of 4 bottles, each for a 6 hour collection, to commence when symptoms appear; this would apply particularly to VMA and catecholamine tests, in which high concentrations may be excreted over short periods of time.

FAECES

Small faecal samples

These are required for such purposes as occult blood detection, inspection for fat globules or porphyrin analysis, and may simply be collected by using a spatula to transfer the sample into a polythene container.

Whole stool samples

These are required over a period of days for faecal fat analysis, in which case a 5 day collection is preferable to one over a shorter period. The whole sample may be taken from a bedpan lined with cellophane, and placed in a plastic carton, with the date and time of the specimen carefully noted, in addition to the patient's name and hospital number. If a marker such as carmine or chromium sesquioxide has been used, specimens both before and after the complete passage of the marker are also necessary, in order to ensure accuracy. It is important in the performance of balance studies for the patient to pass motions regularly and without the use of laxatives, though if these are required the laboratory must be informed. The patient should be given a high roughage diet; normal exercise is encouraged within the limits of the cardiac and respiratory systems in order to maintain regular bowel habits.

SPECIMEN HANDLING AND TRANSPORTATION

Specimens should be transported in safety bags, together with appropriate hazard warnings regarding hepatitis B, HIV-positivity and AIDS (when known), radioactivity and other risks, to the appropriate laboratory without delay. Blood samples should be carried, held vertically in special trays, and delivered to the receptionist in the laboratory. Samples should not be placed unattended near radiators or left on a bench in the laboratory. In the case of emergency samples, the appropriate biochemist or medical laboratory scientific officer should have been contacted in advance; again, the samples must be transported without delay, in this case personally to the analyst concerned.

In a number of instances, special transportation of a particular specimen to the laboratory will be necessary in order to prevent untoward changes occurring with time. For example, some samples require to be transported without delay on ice, in order to permit rapid centrifugation for separation of cells from plasma and immediate storage of the frozen specimen. Any specimens likely to be required for medico-legal purposes must be transported under strict conditions in which proof of identity can be confirmed. Specimens for more than one laboratory should be collected and transported separately to the appropriate laboratories. Attention must be paid to local postal regulations.

APPENDIX III
SPECIMEN COLLECTION, HANDLING AND
TRANSPORTATION - SPECIFIC DETAILS*

BLOOD

Adrenocorticotrophic hormone (ACTH)

Venous blood (20 ml) is collected with a polythene syringe and placed into a polythene bottle containing heparin, pre-cooled on ice. It is centrifuged immediately, the plasma being separated into another polythene bottle and frozen at – 20 °C within 20 minutes of collection. The presence of visible haemolysis in the plasma invalidates results. Specimens are transported in the frozen state.

Aldosterone - fasting

The patient should have been lying down for at least 2 hours and should not have been receiving antihypertensive therapy or diuretics for 3 weeks. Venous blood (10 ml) is collected into a polythene bottle containing heparin. After centrifugation, the plasma is separated into a second polythene bottle and frozen immediately at –20 °C.

Ammonia

Venous blood (2 ml) is collected into a special polythene bottle, free of ammonia, containing heparin, pre-cooled on ice and the cells separated without delay in a refrigerated centrifuge. Arterial blood may also be used. The specimen is transported on ice to the laboratory immediately. If the result is within the reference range, the test should be repeated one hour after a high protein/amino acid load.

Blood Gases

Arterial blood (10 ml) is collected in a polythene syringe containing heparin and from which all air has been excluded. The specimen is transported to the laboratory, on ice, in the syringe with a cap fitted to exclude contact with air. Analysis should be carried out within 30 minutes.

*N.B. The local laboratory should be consulted for precise instructions prior to specimen collection; the instructions given here should be regarded as a guide only.

Calcitonin (CT) - fasting

Venous blood (5 ml) is collected in a polythene syringe, and placed into a polythene bottle containing heparin, pre-cooled on ice, and centrifuged immediately. The plasma is separated into a second polythene bottle and frozen at $-20\,°C$ within 10 minutes. The presence of visible haemolysis in the plasma invalidates results.

Catecholamines (Adrenaline and Noradrenaline)

The patient should not have been receiving antihypertensive drugs for one week. Venous blood (10 ml) is collected into glass bottles containing heparin and sent to the laboratory immediately for centrifugation at $+4\,°C$, with the plasma being stored at $-20\,°C$. Further transportation must be with the specimens deep frozen. Analysis should be performed within one week.

Copper

Venous blood (5 ml) is collected into a plain polythene bottle.

Gastrin - fasting

Venous blood (10 ml) is collected into a polythene bottle containing heparin and Trasylol, pre-cooled on ice, and centrifuged immediately. The plasma is separated into another polythene bottle and frozen at $-20\,°C$ within 15 minutes.

Lactate - fasting

Venous blood (approximately 1 ml) is collected without stasis into cooled pre-weighed glass bottles on ice, containing 2 ml of 0.6 M perchloric acid, and thoroughly mixed. The bottles are re-weighed and the exact amount of blood calculated from the difference between the two weights. All weighings should be carried out at room temperature and bottles should not be touched other than by the gloved hand.

Lipoprotein Lipase - fasting

Venous blood (5 ml) is collected from the fasting patient into a glass bottle containing sodium citrate, centrifuged and the plasma stored at $-20\,°C$.

Parathyroid Hormone (PTH) - fasting

Venous blood (10 ml) is collected in a polythene syringe and placed into a plain polythene bottle. After 30 min this is centrifuged and the serum separated into another polythene bottle, which is frozen immediately at – 20 °C and stored for 24 hours before analysis.

Pyruvate - fasting

Venous blood (approximately 1 ml) is collected without stasis into cooled pre-weighed glass bottles containing 2 ml of 0.6 M perchloric acid. The bottles are re-weighed and the exact amount of blood calculated from the difference between the two weights. All weighings should be carried out at room temperature, and bottles should not be touched other than by the gloved hand.

Renin - fasting

The patient should not have been receiving antihypertensive therapy or diuretics for three weeks. Two specimens of blood are required, the first between 8.00 and 9.00 am with the patient lying flat after 8 hours sleep and the second after being in the upright posture and having undergone light exercise for 30 minutes. Venous blood (10 ml) is collected into a polythene bottle containing heparin and centrifuged immediately; the plasma is stored without delay in a second polythene bottle at –20 °C.

Vitamin A - fasting

Venous blood (10 ml), collected in a syringe protected from light by being wrapped in metal foil, is placed in a plain glass bottle, also protected from light.

Zinc - fasting

Venous blood (2 ml) is collected in a specially prepared plain zinc-free polythene bottle, using a polythene syringe and stainless steel needle (not a rubber-containing vacuum tube). Haemolysis invalidates the results. Care should be taken to ensure that neither zinc-containing medications (including zinc insulin preparations), nor topical applications of zinc ointments/creams are being prescribed. After centrifugation, the serum is stored at – 20 °C in a specially prepared acid-washed polythene bottle.

URINE

Aldosterone

A 24 hour urine collection is made into a polythene bottle containing 10 ml 1% boric acid solution as preservative, and sent to the laboratory without delay.

Copper

A 24 hour urine collection is made into a specially prepared polythene bottle, acid-washed to remove traces of copper.

Iron

A 24 hour urine collection is made into an acid-washed iron-free polythene bottle and acidified to pH 2.0

Lead

A 24 hour urine collection is made into a lead-free polythene bottle and acidified to pH 2.0.

Organic Acids

A random urine specimen (10 ml) for estimation of organic acids (including orotic acid) is collected into a plain polythene bottle, well stoppered, frozen immediately and stored at $-20\ ^\circ$C.

pH

A random specimen of urine (5–10 ml) is collected into a plain polythene bottle and the pH measured immediately at room temperature.

Vitamin C

A 24 hour urine collection is made into a dark bottle containing 20 ml glacial acetic acid as preservative. Upon completion, the sample is sent immediately to the laboratory for analysis.

Xanthurenic Acid

A 24 hour urine collection is made into a polythene bottle containing 2 ml toluene as preservative. The specimen is sent to the laboratory immediately upon completion of the collection. An aliquot is taken and frozen at – 20 °C and the total urine volume measured.

Zinc

A 24 hour urine collection is made into a specially prepared acid-washed zinc-free polythene bottle and stored at +4 °C. Care should be taken to ensure that neither zinc-containing medications (including zinc insulin preparations) nor topical applications of zinc ointments/creams are being prescribed.

APPENDIX IV
TABLE

Base-line plasma/serum hormone concentrations and responses to stimuli in the 'Hypothalamic-pituitary (anterior) function (combined hypothalamic-releasing hormone/insulin) test' (see page 88), 'Insulin stress test' for hypothalamic-pituitary (anterior) assessment (see page 91) and 'Pituitary (anterior) function (combined hypothalamic-releasing hormone/arginine vasopressin) test' (see page 123).

HORMONE		BASE-LINE VALUE	PEAK VALUE	CHANGE IN VALUE
ACTH		<80 ng/L	up to 1000 ng/L	>10 times base-line value
GH		<10 mIU/L	20–70 mIU/L	>2 times base-line value
Cortisol		140–640 nmol/L	540–785 nmol/L	>170 nmol/L
LH*		3–10 IU/L	10–40 IU/L	>2 times base-line value
FSH*		1.5–6 IU/L	5–35 IU/L	>2 times base-line value
TSH		<7 mIU/L	5–25 mIU/L	>5 times base-line value falling with age, but not <2 times base-line value
PRL	M	3–178 U/L	>400 U/L	>3 times base-line value
	F	25–396 U/L	>800 U/L	>6 times base-line value

*These figures are not applicable to the ovulatory phase in females, nor after the menopause.

REFERENCES

1. Kay, J.D.S., Oberholzer, V.G., Seakins, J.W.T. and Hjelm, M. (1987). Effect of partial ornithine carbamoyltransferase deficiency on urea synthesis and related biochemical events. *Clin. Sci.*, **72**, 187–193

2. Elliot, S. and Vessel, M.D. (1979). The antipyrine test in clinical pharmacology: conceptions and misconceptions. *Clin. Pharm. Ther.*, **26**, no 3, 275–286.

3. Fromm, H. and Hofmann, A.F. (1971). Breath test for altered bile-acid metabolism. *Lancet*, **2**, 621–625.

4. Trimble, M.R. (1988). Affective disorders. In Trimble, M.R. *Biological Psychiatry*, Ch. 9, pp. 241–282. (Chichester, New York, Brisbane, Toronto, Singapore: John Wiley and Sons).

5. Pancreolauryl test (fluorescein dilaurate and fluorescein sodium): a routine test for the assessment of exocrine pancreatic digestive function. International Laboratories Limited, Wilsom Road, Alton, Hampshire, GU34 2TJ.

6. Marks, V. and Marrack, D. (1962). Glucose assimilation in hyperinsulinism. A critical evaluation of the intravenous glucose tolerance test. *Clin. Sci.*, **23**, 103–113.

7. Corbett, C.L., Thomas, S., Read, N.W., Hobson, N., Bergman, I. and Holdsworth, C.D. (1981). Electrochemical detector for breath hydrogen determination: measurement of small bowel transit time in normal subjects and patients with the irritable bowel syndrome. *Gut*, **22**, 836–840.

8. Cook, H.B., Lennard-Jones, J.E., Sherif, S.M. and Wiggins, H.S. (1967). Measurement of tryptic activity in intestinal juice as a diagnostic test of pancreatic disease. *Gut*, **8**, 408–414.

9. Holbrook, I.B. (1988). Gastrointestinal tract function tests. In Gowenlock, A.H., McMurray, J.R. and McLauchlan, D.M. (eds.) *Varley's Practical Clinical Biochemistry*, 6th Edition, Ch 27, pp. 670–714. (London: Heinemann Medical Books).

10. Brown, M.J., Alison, D.J., Jenner, D.A., Lewis, P.J. and Dollery, C.T. (1981). Increased sensitivity and accuracy of phaeochromocytoma diagnosis achieved by use of plasma-adrenaline estimations and a pentolinium suppression test. *Lancet*, **1**, 174–177.

11. Sandler, L.M., Burrin, J.M., Joplin, G.F. and Bloom, S.R. (1986). Combined use of vasopressin and synthetic hypothalamic releasing factors as a new test of anterior pituitary function. *Br. Med. J.*, **292**, 511–514.

References

12. Hjelm, M., Brown, P. and Briddon, A. (1986). Sweat sodium related to amount of sweat after sweat test in children with and without cystic fibrosis. *Acta Paediatr. Scand.*, 75, 652–656.

13. Dicopac: A dual isotope test for vitamin B_{12} malabsorption. Amersham International plc, Lincoln Place, Green End, Aylesbury, Buckinghamshire, HP2O 2TP.

INDEX

All the function tests which are referred to in the text commence with a capital letter; in addition, those dealt with in special detail appear in bold type. Also in bold type, but commencing with a lower case letter, are the names of drugs used in the tests, compounds administered and procedures involved.

Figures in bold type represent the main reference pages for the above groups, and the main headings of Appendix I (Preparation of the patient and patient after-care), Appendix II (Specimen collection, handling and transportation – general principles), Appendix III (Specimen collection, handling and transportation – specific details) and Appendix IV (Table).

191

199